MEDIC 16, MEDIC 16
Chronicles of a Street Medic

by

Mark Praschak

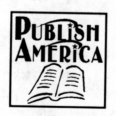

PublishAmerica
Baltimore

First printing

ISBN: 1-60813-219-6 (softcover)
ISBN: 978-1-4489-1735-8 (hardcover)
PUBLISHED BY PUBLISHAMERICA, LLLP
www.publishamerica.com
Baltimore

Printed in the United States of America

Table of Contents

Chapter 1: The Beginning, of Course 7
Chapter 2: The Ambulance 11
Chapter 3: Lost and Found 15
Chapter 4: Back to the Journey 20
Chapter 5: Welcome to the Jungle, Baby 24
Chapter 6: The Knife and Gun Club 34
Chapter 7: Welcome to the World 44
Chapter 8: What's Wrong with This Picture? 50
Chapter 9: It Is What It Is 62
Chapter 10: Them Changes 70
Chapter 11: Welcome, Rookie 79
Chapter 12: Boot Camp 93
Chapter 13: Perseverance 107
Chapter 14: A Higher Power 120
Chapter 15: Once a Grunt, Always a Grunt 130
Chapter 16: The "Little Jake" 143
Chapter 17: Heroes 161
Chapter 18: The Beginning of the End 180
Epilogue 196

Memorial

This book is dedicated to the men and women of Emergency Services and their families, worldwide. It's written for and about those who serve, protect, and put their own lives on the line for people they don't even know, every day.

On September 11, 2001, the World Trade Center attack made everyone in the world understand what dangers Emergency Services personnel face on a daily basis. It's a shame that it took a heinous act of terrorism and the largest single incident loss of life that any fire department or police department had ever encountered to open people's eyes to the reality that surrounds them.

More than any one person, or persons, this book is written in memory of those brothers and sisters that made the supreme sacrifice on that horrific day in September, and for every other being, in every department large or small, who has given his or her life in the line of duty. We know exactly what they're all doing right now; they're protecting the house of God.

I'd like to thank my mom, whom I lost suddenly in August of 2000, my dad and family, and my friends for supporting me throughout my career. I entitled the book *Medic 16, Medic 16* because that was the one radio transmission I heard more than any other over the years. I learned to dread it. I was a career paramedic firefighter for over twenty years and this is my story.

Chapter 1
The Beginning, of Course

It was a frigid Sunday morning when the Claxon horn at the station blared, and the alert tone made me jump out of my skin. We had just received a call for an apartment fire at the garden apartments down the road. Was it a pot of food or steam from a dryer vent? Would I have to make a rescue? My mind and heart were racing. Doug, who lived next door to the firehouse, had the newer of our two pumpers fired up in what seemed like seconds. Louie, who lived two blocks up Main Street, *ran* to the firehouse for calls often, and had just blasted through the front door. My friend Steve and I were in turnout gear in a flash. Doug, who was the senior member, told me to ride the back step in case we needed to lead off (lay a hose line from the hydrant to the fire). My heart was beating faster than the Mack pumper's motor was running, and I was on the step, *alone*.

The four of us screamed down Main Street, siren and air horns blaring. Sunday morning made for very little traffic and I had a death grip on the grab bar and side handle. As we made the turn onto Chartley Drive we saw a column of smoke and fire coming from the third floor apartment. Shit, why couldn't it be the first floor? Dragging 250 feet of two-and-a-half-inch hose filled with water (called the blitz line) up three stories is a ball buster. It was named that because of its potential to put a lot of water on a fire in a short period of time. We hit the hydrant (hooked up to it) and laid a supply line to the fire. After getting the signal from Doug, I opened the hydrant and charged the supply line, then ran to the engine to mask up (put on an SCBA or self-contained breathing apparatus). I would back up Steve and Louie, who were working hard to get the blitz line up the stairs.

Doug was the driver and pump operator. He had to stay with the engine at all times to assure we had water and communicate with the other equipment coming to assist us. I climbed the steps and found Steve and Louie getting ready to make entry into the apartment. It was hot and smoke was banked down practically to the floor. I was sucking up a lot of air from my mask after the run and the climb up the stairs with fifty pounds of gear on. Steve was on the nozzle and looked over his shoulder to make sure Louie and I were in position and ready to go. He reached up and opened the door. The fire immediately roared over our heads.

In a split second, Steve dropped the nozzle and was climbing over us, screaming. Something happened to him. He must have gotten burned or something. Louie took over on the nozzle with me as his backup. He opened up the nozzle as we entered, dragging what felt like a ton of hose into the apartment. He rotated it in a circular motion just like we were taught. It was *really* hot now; steaming hot from the cold water blasting into the inferno. It was hotter than any fire I had felt at the training academy. We inched our way further into the apartment with the nozzle flying. Suddenly, it got dark and I knew that that was a beautiful thing.

We had gotten to the seat of the fire and knocked it down. In other words, we had the upper hand. I felt someone push up against me from behind and a hand on my shoulder. I had someone backing me up me now, which was a great feeling. After what seemed like an hour, we could start to see things in the apartment. We were actually only ten minutes into the entire operation. I could see daylight through what once was a sliding door to the balcony. The glass was gone and so was most of the wooden balcony. I was glad we didn't have to step outside.

Two more hands came in and Louie and I were out of air. They relieved us and we knew the hard part was over. The two us came trudging away from the building like warriors from a battle, I imagined. Our turnout gear was dripping wet and blackened with soot. Steve was on a stretcher near our ambulance. He had taken burns to his ears and had wet compresses on them. He was alright, just blistered. That had to be a painful thing; just think about it. Louie and I walked back to the engine in search of the water cooler. We took turns refilling our small, Dixie-sized, cups. Doug had a mile-wide grin on his face as he looked at us from his post at the pump panel. He knew we had gotten the job done and knew it was my first. Louie, who rarely used a foul word, looked me in the eye.

"Fuckin-A, brother," he said. That's exactly what we had become— brothers. A bond had just been created between the two of us. Our lives depended on each other and we did what was necessary to take care of each other. We came, we saw, and we kicked ass. It was a feeling that I had never felt before, almost like an adrenaline high. I had just been to a place that regular, everyday people would never go, and probably never wanted to go. I just took a trip to hell and kicked the devil's ass. I was a firefighter and Louie knew it; so did I. I didn't realize it at the time, but Louie would become the person that made me the firefighter that I am today. Any firefighter, whether career or volunteer, will tell you, you'll *always* remember your first job (working fire). I remember mine like it was yesterday.

Like any normal fourteen-year-old, I schemed at ways to get out of the house. One day, a classmate of mine was talking about the junior fire company at our local volunteer fire department in rural Baltimore County. He was a member and was gloating about the activities around the firehouse and how cool it was to go there with his big brother, who was a full-fledged "volly" (volunteer).

Basically, a junior would just do inane stuff around the firehouse like housework, washing vehicles, and would occasionally get to go to a big fire. At the big fires they would get to do inane stuff like rack clean hose back on the engines, help gather up equipment from the fireground, or roll up dirty hose lines, but no real firefighting yet. The best part of it was learning the way of the fire department world. The juniors were always invited to Sunday training sessions, house burnings, and they occasionally got to play cards with the big boys if they needed a third or fourth head. It sounded like fun and was a legit reason to get out of the house, so I joined. My mom was excited.

It was 1969 and the country was imbedded in Viet Nam. Kids my age were doing one of two things—smoking dope and watching their big brothers and sisters protest the war, or trying to carry on a normal life and understand what the war was all about and when it would all be over. I chose the latter. As a freshman in high school I soon learned that peer groups were divided into categories—jocks, nerds, heads (anyone with shoulder-length hair, black tee shirts, bellbottom jeans, and red eyes), motorheads (auto shop students that all drove something with more than 350 horsepower) and the fireheads: us. I was really starting to like the firehouse and the camaraderie after six months.

There was a smaller volunteer company just north of our town that took members at age sixteen. When most companies required you be eighteen and to live in their immediate neighborhood (their *first due* area) to be a member, this one made an exception. Their only requirements were age sixteen and live in the voting district, which I did. As soon as I turned sixteen, I quit the juniors and joined the *real* fire department. It was 1972.

My new company was a rural company with a sparsely populated first due area made up of mostly thoroughbred horse farms and scattered single family homes. They only ran fifty-two calls a year and, if you do the math, that's one call a week. Oh well, I got to ride on the back step of the fire engine and, more importantly, got the opportunity to take my first firefighting class; the University of Maryland Fire and Rescue Institute's Basic Firefighting Course. The course was eight weeks of everything you needed to know to keep yourself alive on the fireground, or at least have a clue what to do if shit went south. I kicked ass, and graduated near the top of my class.

I was now a real firefighter, but the fifty-two-calls-a-year thing got old fast. I wanted to, as they say in the service, put the wet stuff on the red stuff. I wanted to punch out windows, pull ceilings, chop holes in stuff, cut up cars, and maybe even ride an ambulance. I wanted to do it all and do it now. The University of Maryland had created a firefighting machine. I couldn't wait until I turned eighteen and could go back to my home company where they ran calls and had a gut bucket (ambulance). My application was on their desk the week before I turned eighteen. It was late 1973.

My membership was accepted at the first regular company meeting after my eighteenth birthday. I had only been a true member for a couple days when I saw the envy in the eyes of the junior volunteers. I remembered being in their shoes but felt like I had graduated. I had taken the first step in what would, hopefully one day, become a career. That Sunday morning was my first job, and I proved myself worthy. It was time to find out if I had what it took to make it my life.

Chapter 2
The Ambulance

Since the first day I walked through the door at the station I had a certain curiosity about the ambulance. It wasn't the same as riding the fire engine, squad, or brush truck. It was different and so were the stories I heard. It was the only piece you rode where you primarily dealt with *people* that were distressed, and not their *property*. It ran twice as many calls as the engine and squad combined.

Nowadays, fire equipment is dispatched as *first responders,* which are the closest units to a call, or when the closest units that are regularly dispatched are not available. Most have firefighters trained in basic life support (EMT-B's) and BLS equipment on board. Riding the ambulance makes you the *primary* caregivers. I wanted to try it and I still wanted to do it all. It was a few months since I had my first job and Louie had taken me under his wing, so to speak. He knew all the equipment we carried on the engines and squad and knew how to use it. I think he enjoyed showing off his know-how and it was a great refresher for him. I was like his shadow when he was around, yearning for learning.

I'm sure I was a pain in his ass sometimes but he took it all in stride.

The most important thing he taught me was to *do it all and do it well.* If it had wheels and it's sitting in the firehouse, learn to ride it and be good at it; so I did. It actually became a trait of mine. I felt pretty good when Louie asked if I wanted to ride the ambulance with him and his partner Dave as the third person on Sunday nights. Everyone that rode the ambulance regularly had a duty night. That was the night you slept in at the firehouse (or ran down the street in Louie's case). There were some in the company that absolutely refused to ride the ambulance or have anything to do with it and, trust me, that will be a chapter in itself later. I had taken the American Red Cross' Basic First Aid Course while in the junior volunteers and that's all I needed to ride the ambo as third man. Louie and Dave were EMT-A's or Emergency Medical Technician-Ambulance. It was the first, real, nationally accredited basic medical training for field providers and the company rules stated you had to be an EMT-A to drive or be second man (aidman) on the ambulance. Louie wanted to see if I had what it took to be one of them, too. I emulated this guy.

There are several levels of EMT today. An EMT-A *then,* is now an EMT-B or Basic. An EMT-I is an Intermediate and can do limited advance life support skills. An EMT-P is a full-fledged Paramedic and can do every advanced life support skill known to man or allowed by their respective state protocols. Before I get into this too far, let me clarify a few things because lay persons get this screwed up all the time.

When I refer to an *engine* or fire engine, I'm talking about a pumper. It carries 500 to 1,500 gallons of water and a lot of different sized hose lines. *It is not a fire truck.* A fire *truck* refers to a ladder truck, called a hook and ladder in the old days. It has the big, motorized ladder for reaching heights and a truckie's job is different than a firefighter's on an engine company. A truckie will perform rescues and ventilation, open roofs, perform extrications and lighting duties in unison with the engine company who performs the primary attack on the fire. They do salvage and overhaul, which is preserving what's left during the fire and after the fire is out, and "mopping up" any hot spots that are left. A rescue truck or squad is just that. The best way to describe a squad is a truck company without the ladder. It's like a giant toolbox. Their crew does the same job as a truck crew, basically, but a squad normally carries more technical entry and rescue equipment. Brush trucks are four-wheel-drive units that carry lesser amounts of hose and water to add to their mobility off-road. They may be mini-pumpers, converted pickup trucks, or Jeeps. Now that we have that cleared up, back to the story.

Dave and I lived too far from the firehouse to run so we slept in on Sunday nights. Unlike my first real fire, I can't tell you what my first ambo call was. There have been too many. I *can* remember my first dead person, my first maternity, and my first fire fatality, but all the rest are blended into the past. The *first* dead person I encountered was on the *second* Sunday that I rode as the *third* man. It was an auto accident where a car left the road and rolled over, just once, judging from the damage. It was on its wheels when we got there and there was very little crush damage to the roof. The sad and sickening part of it was, the driver wasn't wearing his seat belt and was partially ejected through the driver's window when it rolled. He was dead; flattened like a pancake from the waist up including his head, which made for a nasty mess.

This was the first time I'd seen a truly dead person and I realized how important a seat belt really is. It seemed surreal to me. I think if he'd have been belted, he'd have probably been standing next to his car waiting for us to get there. Louie had asked me to get a blanket and sheet from the ambo. When I returned, he opened the blanket and put it partially under the driver's door. Dave simply pulled the door handle, opened the door, and let the lifeless body slip onto it. Then they dragged the blanket away from the car and used the sheet to cover the gore. I wasn't sick but was chilled at the ease of my crew's action and the new smell I encountered—the smell of brain matter. Like burnt flesh or hair, it's a smell like no other and one that I would not soon forget. It seemed as though Louie and Dave had done this a hundred times before. There was no emotion, no comments or anything.

Another first encounter on this call was a thing known as bystanders. It was around midnight on Sunday and I was amazed at the number of people who had gathered, inching their way closer and closer to the scene. Louie shouted at them to back up. They moved a few feet back and he just looked at me and shook his head. We were waiting for the Medical Examiner and our squad to arrive. The squad would set up floodlights so the police could do their accident investigation, which is SOP (standard operating procedure) for any fatal or near-fatal accident. The ME would pronounce the victim dead, then we could remove the body from the scene. A half an hour after the squad had the scene lit the ME arrived. We moved towards the corpse and so did the bystanders. The ME walked up, threw the sheet off the body, and turned to the crowd.

"Is this what you wanted to see?" he asked them.

I've never seen anything like it before. Half of them turned and ran and the other half just started walking away. One of them was heaving like he was going to blow dinner. I guess that's what they wanted to see but I didn't, and still don't, understand. People's affinity with gore and mutilation just doesn't make sense to me. I've learned that this is all part of the scenario and you have to deal with them.

After six months of Sunday nights, I proved to be a worthy member of the crew. I took EMT-A and passed with flying colors. I was cleared to ride as the aidman and eventually drive. Louie and I became the Sunday night crew when Dave's marriage went sour and he started drinking a lot. Once again, it was Louie who taught me how to deal with the job at hand. The joy, sadness, and all the other emotions you encountered on every call were real, and *you better know how to deal with your own emotions before you try to deal with someone else's.* It was 1974 and I was learning about life and death.

Chapter 3
Lost and Found

When I was old enough to push a lawnmower without hurting myself (I think I was four), I got my first job. I would go around the neighborhood looking for lawns that needed to be mowed. Mind you, not ones that needed farm equipment to cut them. I found a little old lady who lived by herself and needed someone to take care of her lawn on a regular basis. I was set.

Later, during high school, I worked pumping gas and doing service station work, cleaning the shitters, and sweeping up after the mechanics. I was saving for a car but wasn't allowed to have one before I graduated, like a lot of my friends did. One day, a couple of months before graduation (and my parents were *sure* I was going to graduate), they let me buy a car. It was a '63 Volkswagen Beetle that had faded, dark green paint and rust holes in the body, but it ran and was only $300. Then $258 later, it passed state inspection. It was a piece of junk. I got an Earl Sheibe $49.95 paint job (that cost $149.00 after the rust holes were patched), and threw a hunk of green shag carpet in it. I suddenly realized where the saying "You can't polish a turd" came from. At least I had my independence.

I graduated from high school in June of 1973 and was the proud recipient of a State Senatorial Scholarship. It paid my tuition to the local community college for two years. I was happy living with my parents, working at the gas station, and going to school where I was majoring in Fire Service Technology; what else? This didn't leave much time for the firehouse and I became, basically, inactive except for the monthly meetings and an occasional call on the weekends. I had my sights set on becoming a paid man (career firefighter).

One day, in October of 1974, I came home from school to find my mom bubbling over. My dad had just gotten a promotion. He worked as a loss control specialist for an insurance company in Baltimore and was promoted to manager. This was a *big* promotion and meant that we had to relocate to

Cincinnati. *Cincinnati? No way, not me.* No crab cakes, Ocean City, Chesapeake Bay, Orioles, Colts, or Natty Boh (National Bohemian, a cat-piss-like beer that was brewed in Baltimore)? I was devastated but, more importantly, I was staying put.

This was my home and the decision was all mine. Little did I know then, but I was about to pull into the fast lane of life. No question, there were things I needed. I innocently learned about Maslow's Hierarchy Theory—food, clothing, shelter, and gas money. I needed a full-time job, some *reliable* transportation, and a roof over my head. There were no relatives to mooch from now, I was on my own. I wasn't leaving the nest, the nest was leaving me.

Dad cashed in a couple of chips at work and got me a good job at a sand and gravel company, about forty miles south of Baltimore. I'd be working as a dispatcher in a scale house, taking orders and coordinating the delivery of sand and gravel to contractors and customers. It wasn't the career I had planned but the pay was pretty good and I'd be able to support myself. With all that said, I bought a new car and found a cheap apartment in Anne Arundel County, closer to the plant. For the next six years there would be no firehouse. It was a time in my life that I look back on and wonder how I survived.

These were truly fast times where fast cars, fast women, facial hair, and an excessive amount of partying were the order. As I look back, I realize how lucky I am today. I was living very close to the edge back then and didn't give a rat's ass about anything. I was pretty popular with my newfound friends, too. I had a hot car, which meant I had hot women, and I was the last of the big spenders especially after Grandpa died and left me $23,000. It was no wonder I was so popular. I was back to living from paycheck to paycheck, six months later.

One night, while hanging out at the car wash (if you had a hot car, you had to hang at the car wash), we saw the local fire engine and ambulance hauling ass down the road. A friend of mine jumped in the car with me and we followed them, just for something to do. We found the call. It was a crash at the intersection of the main highway in town and State Route 3, which is a four-lane divided highway. It was an ugly crash, too.

A car heading south on Route 3 had run a red light and was jammed under a flatbed tractor-trailer. The roof was sheared off the car and it was, actually, completely under the trailer. We parked out of the way and I ran to the scene, as my friend walked. There were four people in the car; two were pinned, and two were lying on the highway. The pinned driver was decapitated. A rear-seat passenger was alive but critically injured, as were the two on the street. I guessed that they were able to crawl out. I immediately identified myself as a provider to the guys on the ambulance.

"Pick one!" they shouted. I ran to the back of the ambulance and grabbed a handful of trauma pads, gauze pads, roller bandages, a cervical collar, and went to the first victim I came to. He and the other passenger in the car were a short distance from the wreckage. I didn't know what it was then, but he had a LaForte 4 fracture, which is a massive fracture of your major facial bones. It's usually a depressed fracture of the face and this one surely was. I was afraid he was going to *code* (a term used for cardiac arrest or short for *Code Blue*, a hospital term). I quickly slipped the collar on him and rolled him up on his side, supporting his head with one hand and his back with my knees. I grabbed a trauma pad with my free hand and ripped the plastic wrapper off with my teeth. I was trying to keep his airway from filling up with blood. One of the first things you're taught in any CPR or first aid class is the ABC's—airway, breathing, and circulation. If you take away any one, you die. This guy had aspirated blood (got blood in his lungs) and probably had a chest injury to boot. I didn't have a chance to look yet because, right now, I wasn't getting past the "A" part of the ABC's. He was gurgling, but still breathing. I knew, then, where the phrase "up to your ass in alligators" came from because I was there.

After what seemed like an eternity, a county paramedic unit rolled up and one of the medics came to help me. I gave him a quick summary and, of course, he could see it wasn't pretty. He was a career *Glitter Boy* (term we used for a Nationally Registered EMT-Paramedic; their patches have gold threads sewn in them that actually make them glitter) and we both knew that this guy's chances of survival were slim, but we pressed on. The medic got a suction unit and a backboard and straps, as we both worked to keep this guy breathing.

I heard a helicopter overhead and then, *NightSun*. It's the biggest remote-control flashlight known to man and is mounted on the belly of the Maryland State Police med-evac helicopter. They were going to land at the scene since the highway was completely shut down. The happiness I felt, that I could actually see what I was doing, quickly turned into anger when I noticed I was kneeling in a pool of clotted blood. Oh well, it was too late to worry about it now.

I figured that all three victims were going to fly by med-evac to the Shock Trauma Center in Baltimore, unless one of the others had coded, then they would go by land to the closest hospital that was fifteen minutes up the road. The flight medic came to us first because we were closest. He took a quick look and said he'd be right back as he headed for the car. We had finished securing the victim to the board and the medic had two IV's running wide open to try and maintain the guy's blood pressure.

The flight medic returned and said he could take both victims. The passenger that was pinned had "coded" and was still pinned. I heard the familiar sound of the Hurst tool (Jaws of Life) generator running. It was a sound that I associated with impending death for some poor soul. When you have an extended extrication time and a trauma patient goes into cardiac arrest you X him off (consider him dead). The chances for survival after cardiac arrest due to trauma, or trauma arrest, are slim to none and less than that if you can't do effective CPR and can't remove the victim quickly, or "load and go."

We carried our patient to the waiting helicopter and walked back to the scene. Their second patient was loaded and they lifted off. Shock Trauma at the University of Maryland Hospital (we called it *Shock-A-Rama*) in Baltimore was only about six minutes away by air. I stopped, took a deep breath, and looked at the carnage around me. Then, I tried to recall what had just occurred. It was then that I realized what had happened.

Every move that I had made, every thought that I had came naturally like breathing. I worked like a machine programmed to do a job. I thought back to the night of my first fatal when I watched Louie and Dave move effortlessly through that call. I realized *who* I was and *what* the gods had meant for me to do. I was a put here, on this rock, to be a *medic*. I walked back to the ambulance to clean up. I was wearing shorts and had blood on my knees and splashes on my arm. The medic I was working with approached me.

"Nice job back there," he said. I thanked him and he asked me if I was in the service (fire department). I made a long story short and shook my head.

"Maybe again, some day," I replied. He told me that the vollies, that were there, were pretty good, and had the only volunteer paramedic unit in the county, that I should think about it. I thanked him again and did what he suggested.

Two days later I got a haircut, shaved my face (except for my mustache), and went to the local firehouse for an application. I had wasted away for six years. I was wild, reckless, and irresponsible, and my future was day-to-day. I made up my mind that night, I had to change. It was the summer of 1980 and time to get back on the track.

Chapter 4
Back to the Journey

The volunteer fire company in Anne Arundel County was different than the one I had come from in Baltimore County. The main drag (literally) where the station was situated was a four-lane highway that passed in front of a four-bay brick building with a banquet hall, large bunkroom, kitchen, shower, and huge TV room. It was pretty classy compared to the small old building on Main Street where I had started out.

I dropped my application off and was told that I would have to wait until the monthly meeting was held, and that I should be present that night. They called me the next week and I arrived early the night of the meeting. I got a pretty cold reception. I guess it was an initiation or something because no one spoke to me; not a *Hi, who the hell are you?* or anything. I was cool and went out into the engine room to look over the equipment. I was pretty impressed and excited at the same time—two Seagrave engines (one brand new), a Jeep CJ5 brush vehicle, a retired military Jeep Comanche that had been converted into a brush truck, a Chevy box-type ambulance, and a Ford Galaxy 500 station wagon, equipped as a paramedic unit.

At seven, people started walking back into the banquet hall where the monthly membership meeting was held. I waited until the hallway was clear then sauntered in and sat in the back of the room, alone. The meeting was called to order and the first order of business was for the membership committee to escort me out of the main hall to the boardroom and give me an oral interview. They were nice to me, I guessed because they had to talk to me. They asked me about my experience, where I worked and my duties there, and some other personal questions, but nothing that made me stop and think. I tried not to be too cocky because I didn't want to come off like that. After the interview, which lasted about twenty minutes, they left and told me to hang tight. They would give the membership their recommendation then vote whether or not to have me. I sat there for ten minutes or so before the chairman of the committee came in, congratulated me, and told me to come join the meeting. I followed him into the hall. He stopped, interrupted the meeting, and introduced me. The president welcomed me and introduced the chief. I would have to talk to the chief about getting my turnout gear and a locker assigned, then I'd be set. I already met the company's requirements to ride the engine and brush trucks but had to take an EMT refresher because my card had expired.

I sat in my original seat by myself and heard some whispers by some of the guys in the crowd, followed by laughter. I was the new guy (aka, FNG) and there was nothing I could do about that. I did know one thing they didn't know yet. I knew I was a good firefighter and EMT and I'd just have to make the grade again.

After the meeting I helped myself to some cold cuts and a beer and met Mel. He was the first one to break the ice. He was one of the guys on the ambo the night of the nasty crash and recognized me. We talked for a while, then went into the engine room and found an empty locker and spare turnout gear that fit me. Mel seemed like a nice guy and asked me when I'd be around. I told him I worked every weekday but would be around on Saturday. He said he'd be there too, and I felt good.

I walked into the kitchen of the firehouse that Saturday morning at around eleven. There were six or eight vollies and three paid men. The paid men were assigned to work at this particular station which was new to me. Anne Arundel County had a combination department, which meant they had career firefighters in all of the twenty-nine volunteer stations to supplement staffing. This was helpful during the day when volunteers were working their regular jobs and at a premium, or at companies where volly membership was low. The three at this station were a driver, or engineman, and two firefighter EMT's.

Three of the vollies were working on a jigsaw puzzle and the others were in the TV room. Once again it was a cold reception. Mel wasn't there yet and I was the new guy again. I sat and watched them try to put this puzzle together. It was like watching paint dry. I saw a piece that fit. Should I ask first or just go for it? Hell, you know what I did. I reached across in front of the biggest guy and clicked the piece in place. All three of them looked up at me.

"What?" I said, with a big, shit-eating grin.

The big guy, named Rex, barked out, "What's your name, Praycheck?"

I barked right back, "It's Praschak." (pronounced praz-chek).
"Praycheck, Paycheck, whatever," he said.

One thing I noticed from the first day I joined the junior volunteers was that everyone in the fire department acquired a nickname sooner or later, even the paid men. Thus, I was dubbed, *Paycheck.* In a matter of fifteen minutes, I felt like I had become the newest member of a very special group. I hate jigsaw puzzles, they give me a headache. This one gave me a life. By the way, I worked the puzzle with them for a half hour, until I got a headache, and never found another piece that fit. Mel arrived a short time later and sat down at the kitchen table with me.

"Anybody take you over the engine yet?" he asked.

"Nah, just hangin' out," I said.

"Let's do it," he ordered. We went out into the engine room and he started opening all the compartments on one of the engines.

"Look these over and when you can tell me what's in each one, I'll get you cleared to ride," he advised. I walked around the engine, closing each compartment door I came to. Mel looked at me like I had two heads. I walked up to the driver's front compartment, pointed to it and said, "Pump Operator's compartment; fittings, double males, double females, cellar nozzle, gated wyes, inch-and-a-half nozzle, two-and-a-half-inch nozzle, stacked tips, spanner wrenches, hydrant wrench, rubber mallet, steamer fittings, and a short shot down below."

I walked up to the driver's side rear compartment, pointed to it and said, "Two Circle D's, cord reel, junction box, smoke ejector, ejector hanger, and a box of pigtails."

Mel was standing there with his jaw hanging open.

"Better close that thing, you might catch a fly," I said.

One by one, I went to each compartment and without even opening them, pointed and called off the contents. What do you think I was doing before the meeting? By the time I finished Mel was shaking his head. He went to Sonny, the career engineman, and told him that I was good to go, if we got a run. Sonny just nodded and, like that, I was cleared to ride.

Mel was certified as a CRT or Cardiac Rescue Technician. It was Maryland's version of paramedic just not as advanced as an EMT-P. EMT-P's are college trained with 1,000 hours of field time and have to pass the National Registry exam. None of the volunteer paramedics were EMT-P's yet. The county had just started putting *their* CRT's through the EMT-P pilot program at the local community college.

Anne Arundel County had ten advanced life support units, or paramedic units, stationed throughout the county. This station had the eleventh and the only one completely staffed by vollies. I thought that was pretty cool. The career paramedics were held pretty highly in the service. They were doing *new* things to save lives. A paid man worked a twenty-four-hour shift; on twenty-four hours and then forty-eight hours off. They worked every third day, basically. Their shift started at seven in the morning and ended at seven the following morning. I wondered what that would be like, especially if you were busy all night and didn't get any sack time.

Mel rode the medic unit on Monday nights. He asked me if I liked riding the gut bucket. I said it didn't matter to me, whatever went out the door first. He hinted at me riding the ambulance on Monday nights while he was on the medic unit. I'd think about it and I had just started my EMT refresher course. I was still getting settled in at my new station and didn't want to bite off more than I could chew. After all, I'm the new guy, remember?

After a few months of fire calls and ambo calls, I had established myself as one of the boys. We had jobs, pin jobs (accidents with entrapment), fatals, and big weedbeaters (brush fires). It was the same shit, but in a different place. Eventually, I started to earn some respect. I started riding the ambo on Monday nights while Mel rode the medic unit. I learned, over the next several months, what a great medic he was. Not only was he book-smart, he was great with his skills, and he knew it. Some medics know the books by heart but wouldn't get near me with a needle. No one would ever deny Mel, especially me. We had become good friends and hung out away from the station a lot. I took Mel's advice and applied for the next CRT class.

In July of 1982, I received my Maryland Cardiac Rescue Technician certification thanks to Mel's persistence and a lot of hard work. I'm now a *paramedic* firefighter.

Chapter 5
Welcome to the Jungle, Baby

Being a paramedic in the fire department is special. Its specialized training sets you apart from the others and its duties thrust you into gullet of the animal. It takes you to places you've never been and a lot you never want to return. You know you will, though. Like the first charred body you see that's still alive, or the shotgun blast to the head that doesn't quite get the job done, you know you'll be back and hopefully you'll be better. Does the phrase "Been there, done that" ring a bell?

Mel and I were a great team and I had become as cocky as he was. We were highly respected by everyone in the department, even on the career side. They had seen us work together. When you work side-by-side with someone long enough, you get inside their head and anticipate their every move. That's what a paramedic partnership is: a well-oiled machine. One of you might be better at certain skills. I could start an IV on an ant. Mel did drug dosages in his sleep. We entered the *Emergency Care Skills Competition* sponsored by the Maryland Institute for Emergency Medical Services System, or MIEMSS. Teams from all over the state were there. We posted a third place in 1981(I was still an EMT) and second place in 1982, after I became a CRT. The plaques are *still* in the showcase at the station today. My most treasured memory of the events are a picture of Mel and me with Dr. R. Adams Cowley, the founder of Baltimore's Shock Trauma Center and the *Father of Trauma Care* in this country (if not the world). Baltimore had the first trauma center in the nation.

One of our volunteer paramedics, Kevin, had gotten a job with the Baltimore City Fire Department as a paramedic. He told me that they were always hiring due to a high turnover rate. It was something I'd learn about later. I thought about it long and hard. Should I start there? Anne Arundel County was very particular about who they hired and vollies were considered enemies to the illustrious Firefighter's Union. They still are to this day. Hell, I'm going for it.

On February 10, 1983, I received my letter of acceptance into the Baltimore City Fire Department in the position of Paramedic I. The starting salary was $17,667 per year. The duties were gut bucket only but, hey, I'm a *paid man*. The stories I'm about to tell are true, with a higher power as my witness. The names have been changed to protect the innocent and the mentally challenged.

After a two-week orientation class, I was assigned to Medic 16. It was housed in a station built in 1903 with Engine 1 and Truck 11. There was barely room for all three pieces of equipment but it was very nostalgic. It had brass fire poles. I was gonna have to *slide the pole*. I was afraid to ask for directions on how to do it so I just watched the guy in front of me and hoped for the best. The important thing was to make sure the guy that slides before you is clear and you don't come down on his head. This station was, dead-center in the middle of the city. I was partnered with two African-American individuals that had completed their CRT training through the CETA Job Corp program, sponsored by the department. They were David and Bonnie. David was a five-year veteran and Bonnie had seven years in. There were three of us on a shift because one would, most likely, be off on leave. If all three of us were working, I'd be detailed out to another unit, being the junior man. One thing that did separate us, aside from race, was experience. I came from *the county*. I was seen as a prima donna from day one. The county had nicer equipment, better and more dated toys (radios, EKG monitors, and the like) and fewer calls. These two had no prior experience before CETA. I felt lucky. We worked an unusual shift of four ten-hour days then two days off, followed by four fourteen-hour nights then three days off. The day shift, or *trick*, was bearable but "night tricks" were killer. The paramedics had their own bunkroom but after my first night trick I had to ask myself, *why?* Nine times out of ten, on night work, I'd get to the station at four in the afternoon and wait for the medic unit to return. When it returned, it was in the station for ten to fifteen minutes, at the max, then gone. Out the door we'd go, rarely seen for the rest of the shift. I never imagined running calls non-stop. Oh, we'd make it back to the station on a lot of occasions, but not for long. Even during the day, it was tough to stand in line at McDonald's and get food before getting another call. We were never counted in for lunch or dinner at the station because we were never there. For the first time in my life I understood the meaning of two terms—exhaustion and sleep deprivation. Medic 16 was the seventh busiest unit in the city in 1983, out of sixteen units. They ran 5,600 calls. Medic 7, at the *"Old Town"* station, was the busiest medic unit in the United States that year with over 7,500 calls. I was detailed to Medic 7 more than once. What a freakin' war wagon that was.

I returned to the volunteer station a few times after I got hired but things were different. It was like I had crossed a line that made me different in some way. I could tell by the way that my boys treated me. They all acted pissed off at me. Was it envy or just the harshness of the rivalry between the paid and volunteers in the county that made them act like this? I was confused and hurt. I didn't like it. I felt like I had somehow let them down. The final blow was the day I showed up at the firehouse and was told I couldn't go on a fire call with them so I could *"put the ambulance in service, in case someone else came in while they were gone."* I always rode the first thing out the door unless the engine was full and, only then would I stay back. There was room for me on the step that day, but not with them. I felt abandoned. They had denied me and showed me where they thought I belonged. I left before they returned from the call and never looked back. My days as a volly were over.

I can remember my first call in the city vividly. A sick case outside, always dispatched as "sick on the street." David and I rolled up to find a homeless man sitting in a vacant lot; unusual, you ask? He was a double amputee. He had no legs and was perched on some kind of homemade thing that looked like a small pallet with wheels on it. Being of the homeless breed, referred to by us as *Urban Outdoorsmen,* he was rolling filth. This man actually had insects on him, visible to the naked eye. David chuckled as we loaded him on to the stretcher, pallet and all. He knew I was freaking out. Ah, the smell of year-old body odor and my first encounter with a *Frequent Flyer* (someone who calls for help so much you see them more than some family members).

So this is how you want to make a living, huh? I thought to myself. I worked for the city for about two years. To this day, I describe it as ten years of experience rolled up into two years. I saw things that would amaze you. I started saying, "I've seen it all now" so much that I sounded like a broken record. After a month I realized, I would never see it all. Just when I'd thought I'd seen it all, I'd see something more incredible, or incredibly stupid. I gave up.

Jumpers

I found that people in the city are more creative at committing suicide than their psycho counterparts in the suburbs. I think it has to do with living above sea level in an area that is at sea level. They loved to jump off things, like high rise buildings and bridges. Our radio sounded off.

"Medic 16, Medic 16."

"Medic 16, Brookfield and Whitelock, in service," I answered.

"Medic 16 respond to number 20 East Twenty-First Street for an injured person in front of that address." My first jumper was an obviously distraught young man in his twenties, who decided to pay Grandma a visit at her eighteenth-floor apartment for one reason—to jump off her balcony. It wasn't a pretty sight. As Bonnie and I approached the scene one of the firefighters from 18 Engine (don't ask me why we say it backwards. It's like a NASCAR thing, I think) ran up to us.

"I think he's got a pulse," he said, in a puff. Not knowing the circumstances at the time, we started running toward the patient. I stopped dead in my tracks and stood there gaping when I arrived at the steaming pile of human Jello.

"Where the hell did he jump from?" I shouted.

"The eighteenth floor," the firefighter said quietly.

The man's liver was lying on the sidewalk next to him.

"The only pulse you felt tonight, Bud, was your own. We're outta here," I said, as we left that one for the police and the morgue wagon.

It Was a Perfectly Good Bridge

The alarm sounded five times; we were emptying the house.

"GONG, GONG, GONG, GONG, GONG."

"Engine 1, Truck 11, Medic 16, respond for a report of a person that jumped from the Howard Street Bridge," the house radio sounded. It was a beautiful spring day when we received the call for the jumper from the Howard Street Bridge. It's a bridge about a quarter to a half mile long that crosses railroad tracks, an open area frequented by hobos, and the Jones Falls, a wide-flowing creek that could pass for a small river. Engine 1 went to check out a taxi stopped on the bridge over the tracks; 11 Truck and Medic 16 were directed to Falls Road, under the bridge. We found nothing, but the water was high and flowing rapidly from recent spring rain showers. I was working with Jim, a firefighter detailed from Engine 1 this shift, because both my partners called in sick. Jim liked working with me as opposed to the other two and we eventually became good friends away from the job.

I looked at him and said, "Well, if they jumped here they're at the Inner Harbor by now," considering the speed of the rapidly flowing water. Just then, Engine 1 radioed that a woman was riding in the taxi and shouted "Stop!" just as the taxi entered the bridge. She threw open the door, jumped out of the cab, and over the side of the bridge, without a pause. Didn't have the fare, I guess. The strange thing was, the crew from Engine 1 was looking over the bridge and saw no one. It was about a forty-foot drop. Captain Tom from Engine 1 instructed Truck 11 to go to the Maryland Institute of Art, on one side of the tracks, and Medic 16 to the Community College of Baltimore, on the other side, to see if we could see anything. We did as directed. When the crew from the truck climbed down the embankment to a retaining wall they saw a woman sitting on a large pile of dirt, just under the bridge, smoking a cigarette. They looked over at us and pointed to her. Unbelievable.

The woman hopped out of the cab and off the bridge, landed on her ass on a pile of dirt. She got up, walked under the bridge, climbed up on another pile of dirt, and was having a smoke. She had just left the Psychiatric Unit at University of Maryland Hospital. Escaped would be more like it. We'd stabilize her and drive her to Trauma. Later, we were told she had fractured her sacrum (tailbone).

Choo-Choo's

Jim and I had become a pretty good team together. I got my first Letter of Commendation with him just two months after I got hired.

"Medic 16, Medic 16," the radio blared.

"Medic 16…in service, Saint Paul and Centre Streets," I answered.

"Engine 28, Medic 16 respond to Penn Station, number 1200 Pennsylvania Avenue, for a sick person on an incoming train; ETA fifteen minutes," they ordered. We were working the day shift and got a call to go to the railroad station and stand by for an incoming AMTRAK train with a sick passenger on board. Their ETA was fifteen minutes. Penn Station was two or three minutes away. We were running with Engine 28, but we would get there first. I called them on the radio and told them to have a firefighter help us with equipment. It was a pretty good haul from the street to the loading platform, so we'd take extra things with us. We were set up and ready about five minutes before the train arrived. When the train finally arrived I grabbed my gear bag and oxygen and four of us filed onto the car where the ill person was seated. He was a big, black man, and was *vegged.* That's the term we used for someone that's awake but not responding to your voice or mild painful stimuli, like a pinch. This man was not well.

His breathing was labored, he was drooling, and was incontinent (OK, he pissed himself). Another passenger stated that he just "started snoring," but his eyes were open. They said he didn't have a seizure so right away I'm thinking, diabetic or worse, stroke. We had a device called a stair chair. It's a narrow folding chair with three seat belts and wheels and it's a city paramedic's best friend when it comes to narrow doorways and hallways that are very common in the old row homes.

"We gotta go, bro," I whispered, sharply. Jim sensed the urgency in my words. We got the patient on high-flow oxygen and loaded him up. He had to be six feet, four inches tall and over 250 pounds. There's a fire department formula for people like that. The higher up or the tighter the spot, the bigger they will be. For example, if you go to the lobby of the high rise, the patient will be small. The more floors you have to go up the bigger they will be, especially if it's a building with no elevator.

We got our patient to the medic unit, transferred to the stretcher, and got him as stable as possible with an IV and heart monitor before we headed for the hospital. A few shifts later Jim and I were presented with a letter from the chief of operations from AMTRAK and a letter of commendation from the chief of the fire department, thanking us for a job well done. That made us feel pretty good considering we didn't do anything out of the ordinary for this patient. We recognized the need to load and go and that's what we did. A letter of commendation doesn't come often. We call them *attaboys.* It would be the first of many for me. That doesn't mean I never generated a complaint.

There's one more call that involves a train that comes to mind. David and I were working the night shift on a hot summer night when we got this call.

"Medic 16, Medic 16."

"Medic 16; Moser and McMechon, in service," David returned.

"Medic 16 respond to the Eager Street tunnel for a report of a person lying on the tracks, with Truck 16," the voice commanded.

I had to ask myself, who called this in? It's a train tunnel, not a pedestrian tunnel. Truck 16 would get there first. When they did, they called us and advised that the engineer of a northbound AMTRAK train had entered the tunnel and saw a man lying in between the rails about a quarter of a mile inside the tunnel. He had no chance of stopping and passed over him. The man was located under the third car. Let me tell you something about the Eager Street tunnel. It has two sets of tracks and is about a mile long. It was built back when Jesus was riding trains. One thing I learned is that they don't clean train tunnels—*ever.* Everything we touched inside the tunnel was black with soot from a hundred years of exhaust. I want you to understand what *everything* means. Even the rocks that made up the railroad bed were covered with thick, black powder. We arrived just outside the tunnel entrance with Truck 16.

There was no way to get the ambo into the tunnel so we had to hump all our stuff into this shit hole. I asked the lieutenant from the truck to call for some more hands. Engine 7 was summoned, so we loaded up the stretcher and away we went. Four of us took turns carrying the stretcher loaded with equipment because it was impossible to roll it on the two-inch rocks. Two firefighters from the truck were already tending to the man under the train. Apparently, this gentleman had been drinking and while taking the shortcut home decided to lay down and take a breather, *on the tracks.* Fortunately for him, he was lying between the rails. From my best observation he was lying on his back with one knee up. When the train's locomotive, which has a large I-beam that sticks down and acts like a cow catcher, passed over him, it snapped his leg like a twig. I'll bet if he was lying completely flat, that train would have passed right over him.

Tough break, no pun intended. He had a pretty serious injury. Our mindset was to load him up and get his dumb ass out of there to a better environment where we could better serve him. This was not a patient-friendly place. I have to tell you that the Chessie System guys that were there (they handle freight trains) were on the ball. By the time we had this guy stabilized and out from under the train car, a small yard locomotive had arrived. They told us to lift the patient up and load him on the front of the engine and they'd roll him out for us. Good deal but no easy task. I'm glad the extra hands were there. It took eight of us to lift the 250-plus pounds, ten feet onto the front of that engine.

We "motored" him out and repeated the task of lowering him down and into the medic unit. Of the eight guys there, including myself, three were African-American, but we were all black that night. Everything was covered with soot. I guess it was a blessing in disguise because after we delivered the patient to

Trauma we had a two-hour break getting cleaned up. Gotta take it when you can get it.

Hot Dogs

Domestic disputes are by far the most volatile calls to be on, not just for the police. More police officers are killed in the line of duty on domestics than all other calls combined. They're a load of fun for us, too, especially when we get there *before* the police, and both players are present. The Baltimore Orioles had made the playoffs and a group of friends were having a game party at their row home uptown, when the radio sounded.

"Medic 16, Medic 16."

"Medic 16, Charles and Twenty-Fifth, in service," I chirped.

"Medic 16 respond, 2938 Saint Paul Street, for a person burned with scalding water." Burns are one of the nastiest calls. Whether it's a scald, flames, or anything else, I think if I had to categorize which types of trauma were the worst, burns had to be #1. In our business, it's the one that could kill us at any time. They create an odor that stays with you for hours, and if you know the smell, one that you can detect before you even get to the patient, sort of like hot lead, gunpowder, and brain matter. There will be calls like that later. This particular evening, a young man had apparently made an advance at a young lady at the party. As in most cases, partaking in too much of an alcoholic beverage leads to poor judgment. Too bad for him because *his wife* (who had a nip or two as well) overheard the remarks and promptly went to the kitchen, picked up the large pot of boiling hot dogs, returned, and dumped it over his head. Somehow you knew it was going to leave a mark.

We arrived before the police and found chaos. There were at least twenty people in this little row house and everyone wanted to kick someone's ass (except for two people that were holding a dirty, wet dishtowel over our patient's head). We pushed our way through the mess. I love it when people think we're the police.

"You gotta arrest that fuckin' bitch. She done burned up my boy," one partygoer stated.

"Excuse me, sir, we're not the police, we're the medics, and can you please get the fuck out of our way so we can take care of your boy?"

Ah, if I could just say that to him, but I won't. That would be like pouring gasoline on a fire. Our *boy* had second-degree burns on his head, ears, face, neck, and shoulders, which automatically earned him a free pass to the Baltimore Regional Burn Center at City Hospital, across town. Our first task was to protect him from his *friends* until the police got there. After the police arrived and brought order to the place we quickly shuffled the patient to the ambulance. Some morphine would be in order if we were allowed to carry it (city medic units don't because of the potential for robbery) but I believe this guy had enough liquid painkiller on board before he got splashed. Oh yeah, the Orioles lost 5-3.

Know When to Keep Your Mouth Shut

That story reminded me of a call that almost got me hurt; no fault of mine. I mentioned earlier how some members of the department despised the ambulance and anyone associated with it. It's an *old school* mentality that defines the fire department as just that, the *fire* department. Their mentality was that all ambulances should be run by the hospitals. You found out quickly in each station who the haters were. You'd be called a "street doctor," "nurse" and in some cases, just a "fuckin' paramedic." My all time favorite was "paraqueer." My response to anyone reverting to the name-calling was, "Be thankful I'm doing this fuckin' job, otherwise *you* would be, and you better call me 'sir' when I'm savin' your ass on the fireground." In a lot of cities and towns, ambulances are run by hospitals. Over the years people have become more educated in fire safety, smoke detectors were introduced, and new structures were made more fire resistant, which created a trend of fewer fires each year. Not less calls, though. A lot of departments were losing revenues and downsizing because of this trend and opted to start providing ambulance service to secure funding and staffing. Let me make it clear that some large city departments have provided both for centuries.

I was working with a hater, detailed from 11 Truck, one shift. We'll call him Wigs. Wigs had been a trucky for his entire career, which spanned twenty-plus years. He absolutely hated the ambulance and me, because I worked on it. He drove to calls like a freaking maniac just to try to blow the unit up (like they were going to run out of ambulances and not find some piece-of-crap reserve unit to stick us in). That was my first problem with him. We had words about that on one of our first shifts together, and I actually had to threaten to complain to the company lieutenant just to get him to slow down. What a dumb ass.

We got a call while in the station for an injured person one Sunday afternoon. To compound Wigs' already fine attitude, the call took him away from his football game. I didn't realize watching football was in the job description when I got hired. We hauled ass to this call and I was pissed. As we arrived at the front door of the residence we could hear arguing going on.

"Fire Department!" I shouted, knocking on the door. A female answered the door and I followed. Two males were in the living room, one with a large laceration to his head. All three were high on who knows what.

"You gets to take him to the hospital," the woman shouts. OK, let's clarify something here. Legally, if an adult refuses treatment or transport, we can't treat them and transport them against their own will, drunk or not. That's referred to as *kidnaping*. We can call the police and have them placed in protective custody if they obviously need medical attention and are being irrational, then transport them. Mention the word police to them and one of two things happens—they either run you out of the house, listen to what you have to say, or try to do both. Once again drugs and/or alcohol make for impaired judgment and dull your decision-making skills (if you have any to begin with).

I was able to get this guy's permission to, at least, bandage his head. I was getting tired of waiting for him to pass out from blood loss at which time I would then be bound by law to treat him; no help from Wigs here. He's standing at the door smoking a cigarette like a true professional. After getting the patient's head bandaged, I again pleaded with him to go. It's a bitch trying to get a drunk to go to the hospital when he doesn't want to. It's more of a bitch when two other drunks are trying to *make* you take him. The ultimate bitch is when your so-called partner stands at the door and shouts, "Fuck them, Mark. If they don't want us, let's get the fuck outta here." I happened to be standing between Wigs and the two drunks that wanted to kick both of our asses now. We hit the door running, down the steps and onto the sidewalk where I proceeded to immediately drop my bag. I pushed Wigs up against the ambulance and stuck my finger in his face.

"If you ever open your mouth on another call, you're not gonna have to worry about the family kicking' your ass, motherfucker," I threatened. Understand that Wigs is a big man; much bigger than I am. After I stepped away from him, he didn't move. He leaned up against the ambulance until I finished advising the police that it was a refusal, and told them we were leaving. I thought Wigs' eyes were gonna pop out of his head and I never had a problem with him for the rest of the shift. I'm surprised he didn't claim to be sick when we got back to the station and go home.

Chapter 6
The Knife and Gun Club

In large urban settings, there are elements. Big cities are like a chemical mixing bowl. The mix of certain elements can be lethal. Some of the elements are gambling, prostitution, drugs, alcohol, guns, gang activity, and the list goes on. Most of these are a direct result of poverty and unemployment. Some are a part of organized crime. The violence associated with these elements was simply barbaric acts committed by those seeking revenge, venting anger, collecting debts, or settling a score. In any case, it usually resulted in someone needing me.

I stated earlier that I would have my own opinion about some subjects. I have that right and really don't care if it's the same as yours. You have the same rights. I'm just putting two and two together. In a lot of the cases I handled, which involved shootings, stabs, cuttings, or beatings, it is my belief that the people doing the shooting, stabbing, cutting, or beating couldn't give a rat's ass whether they went to jail or not. Jail or prison was like checking into a cheap hotel to them. They got three squares, room service, uniforms, linens and laundry, gym, basketball, TV, and showers. Most of them didn't have these luxuries on the street, or at home, because they required money, which meant they would have to get a job and work; not likely.

Weekend Fun

Friday and Saturday nights were the busiest time for us, especially at the beginning of the month when welfare and Social Security paid off. Summer was busier because everyone was outdoors. I guess eighty-five degrees outside was better than 110 inside. It didn't matter what time of the year it was when it came to violence. The only difference was, in the winter they would shoot, stab, cut, and beat indoors more.

For those that had jobs, Friday was payday. To this day, I still believe that money makes some people stupid. In some cases *more* stupid than others. People's priorities were all out of whack to me. I like a cold beer now and then, but I have to eat every day. I wouldn't take my whole paycheck and blow it on partying in a week (unless my refrigerator was well stocked and I had gas in my car). I couldn't comprehend this type of behavior.

Getting high or drunk and making a temporary escape from a miserable life is a very popular pastime in the inner cities. The cold, hard facts are when the high or drunk wears off, the misery is still there. Now, not only are you miserable, but broke and miserable. Anger and desperation set in and it all leads to acts of crime and violence. It's sad that I make this sound like the entire population. It's only a small percentage of the population that behave like this, but affects the entire population.

The Knife Club

You don't have to own a knife to be a member of this group. Anything sharp enough to cut or penetrate skin, or scare someone into submission, is suitable. They can be picked up almost anywhere, literally. Scissors, box cutters, razors, razor knives, ice picks, screwdrivers, broken bottles, or even a piece of plate glass with duct tape wrapped around it for a handle, are all you need. Some people should use their creative minds to make a buck instead of being dumb asses. At any rate, I've seen the damage they can do. The radio sounded off.

"Medic 16, Medic 16."

"Medic 16...North and Green mount...in service," I said, in a tired manner.

"Medic 16 respond to the city jail with Truck 16 and Medic 7 for a stabbing with multiple patients," the voice commanded with urgency. This was one place that everyone in the service knew. The dispatcher didn't have to give us the address. I had been on calls to police stations, detention centers, and the Federal prison located in the county. They all paled in comparison to city jail. The place sent cold chills down my spine the first time I went there for a call. Try to picture a 200-year-old, medieval dungeon with modern-day amenities. It even smelled like filth. I hated the place. Just the thought of committing a crime and being sent there was nauseating. Who in their right mind would take that chance? Could this place be better than some people's homes? Maybe, if you lived under a bridge or in a dumpster.

We arrived at the "Sally" port at the facility. A "Sally" port is a series of two fenced gates, exterior, and interior. You enter the exterior gate and it closes behind you and your identifications are checked and vehicle inspected. Then the interior gate opens to give you access to the facility. Yes, even the medic units would get checked (like we were gonna smuggle something in, or maybe someone). Who would want to sneak into this shit hole? I didn't even want to *drive* in on official business. Neither gate can be opened at the same time, to prevent escape. Normally we would enter the port, go through security, and be given directions to the closest access door to the patient. This time it was different. There was a sense of urgency this time. Guards were running around with shotguns, police cars were there with lights flashing, and there was no inspection this time. Usually, the only weapons you see at this place are carried by the tower guards, and are never found on the ground or in the building. As soon as the first gate closed, the second opened. A guard ran up to the driver's side of the unit.

"Follow me," he ordered. David and I just looked at each other. The shit was hitting the fan here and Truck 16 and Medic 7 were already inside. The info we got was that there were three patients. One of them was a guard and a third medic unit was coming. That made it personal now. Even though you think it's just a jail guard, he's still part of the family. They're sworn and dedicated, with a badge and a family, just like us, and a brother or a sister, whether we knew each other or not. That's just the way it is.

Medic 7 called. They were inside and the jail was on "lock-down" (all doors locked). The jail infirmary was bringing our patient out to us. I was happy not to have to go in there. The staff arrived with an inmate on their Gurney, a small man who looked to be thirty or so. It was an easy transfer onto our litter. He was lying face-down and blood stained the back of his shirt. One of the jail staff told us he got a *shank* in the back. A shank is the term used for a homemade knife. It could look like any of the previously mentioned street weapons. The one used today was like an ice pick. After cutting away the inmate's shirt, we started counting wounds. There were seven tiny punctures across his upper back. I suspected he had a lung injury. He was having trouble breathing and his blood pressure was good. It was oxygen, high flow, and time to go.

The one good thing about working in the city was the hospitals. There were dozens of them and most of the time, no matter what section you were in, you weren't far away from one. This guy had gotten a ticket to Johns Hopkins Trauma, which gave me about five minutes to get him on the heart monitor and throw an IV in him (while hauling ass on a downtown street. You should try it sometime). I talked to him to let him know what I was doing and where we were going. I thought about Medic 7 and the guard. I wanted to ask him if he was the perp that stabbed the guard but I didn't. Even if he was, I had my job to do. We got to Hopkins and took the patient to the trauma room. We were waiting for Medic 7 to roll in. They were about two minutes behind us. A few minutes later I heard them coming down the hallway. I was sickened when I heard them, too.

"One, one thousand, two, one thousand, three, one thousand…" Shit. They were doing CPR on the guard as they rolled him down the hall. He was in cardiac arrest.

He succumbed to an injury to his heart a half hour later and *my* heart was hurting. I thought about his family. Did he have kids, a wife, or a mom and dad that was living? Then I got pissed off at the person that did this to him. Was it the guy I just brought in; that fuckin' little punk? I'd let it go because, if I didn't know, I wouldn't do anything stupid. It was on my mind for the rest of the shift. My prayers were with the guard's family because, indirectly, it was my family too. We forgive, but we never forget.

The Gun Club

To be a member of this group you have to be a flat-out, no-holds-barred, out-and-out criminal; period. You've gotten your hands on the deadliest of all weapons. You've either stolen it, bought it on the street, traded drugs or stolen goods for it, or in very rare cases, bought it legally. You don't care about caliber or maintenance, just ammunition. You are the most dangerous of all criminals now. You're a big man even if you're five feet, two inches tall, or thirteen years old. Nobody is going to get in your way, push you around, or talk down to you. Do you have the balls enough to pull the trigger? Of course you do. You think about it all the time. Sometimes you can't wait for the opportunity. Do you care about the person you shoot or their families? Not even after they're dead. You wouldn't have shot him if you did. Do you care about the consequences? You're not smart enough to think that far in advance. As a matter of fact, not only are you the most dangerous, you're in an elite group of criminals—the dumbest.

A Saturday Night Special

Ah, the good old "Special." It's responsible for more misfires than any other firearm, outside of black powder. It's deadly from close range if you're a good shot, or get lucky. This piece is usually twenty-two to thirty-two caliber. In some cases larger caliber, like a Derringer, but they're rarely found on the street. When you buy one on the black market, they're usually old and poorly maintained which accounts for the number of misfires. It's definitely a minor league criminal's weapon, but a gun nonetheless. The radio blared.

"Medic 16, Medic 16."

"Medic 16…clearing Maryland General, in service," I replied.

"Medic 16 respond to The Royal Lounge, 1120 Mount Royal Avenue, for a shooting. Police are en route," the dispatcher said. It was nice of them to let us know that the police were en route to a shooting. Our first due area (which we occasionally saw) had a very diversified mix of customers. We had the Maryland Institute of Art, an exclusive neighborhood called Bolton Hill, the expressway, and to the north, Johns Hopkins University. For reasons not mentioned, we seemed to have a large number of residents that enjoyed the "alternate" lifestyle—homosexuals, bisexuals, cross-dressers, and transvestites. It was too much for me to try to comprehend. The bar we were going to was frequented by those aforementioned type individuals—OK, it was a fag bar, for Christ's sake.

When we arrived the police had secured the scene and we entered the bar to find a man (I think), reportedly the bartender of this fine establishment, sitting on a chair with a towel around his left elbow. He said a guy shot him twice. It was obviously a small-caliber wound. He was up and talking. I removed the towel to find a wound that entered the back of his left upper arm, exited, and went through his left lower arm as well. The shooter had to be pretty close when he popped him. When I attempted to move his arm, he complained of pain in his side. Behold, shot number one went in the side of his lower left chest. Now, we have a problem. Apparently the first shot to the chest made him bend his arm to guard the injury and the second shot went through his bent arm. We moved a little faster now. These are patients that will be talking to you one minute and are in cardiac arrest the next. We got him out to the ambulance and started to work with oxygen, assessment, EKG, IV, and then go. It was pretty standard procedure. Upon further assessment on the way to the hospital, I realized how lucky this guy really was. Oh, by the way, he was a guy. With no real serious bleeding, a normal BP and no trouble breathing, you just have to look again (you should anyway). He had a large mass right above his genital area, in the middle of his lower abdomen.

The small caliber bullet had ricocheted off his left floating rib and lodged right there. It probably didn't travel through anything but fat until it stopped. Count your blessings and stop fooling around with another man's man, Man. OK, I'm done.

Are You Feeling Lucky?

A lot of times our calls would be across town, requiring some time to get there. That being the case one night, we responded from the station to a reported gunshot wound to the head with Engine 58. Whenever we had an extended ETA, the company on the scene would usually call and give us a patient status report. We had a twenty-minute ride to this call.

"Engine 58 to Medic 16," the Officer on engine called. We could hear a ruckus in the background but the voice on the radio was fairly calm.

"Medic 16 to 58, go ahead," I answered.

"We have a twenty-year-old black male with a small caliber gunshot wound to the forehead. He's conscious and alert. What's your ETA?" Did I just hear what I thought I heard?

"Eight minutes, 58. Did you say conscious and alert?" I asked.

"That's correct 16. He's sitting on the steps in front of the residence," he said. David and I just looked at each other and shrugged our shoulders. When we arrived, sure enough, there he sat with a golf ball-sized knot right in the middle of his forehead. He was pissed off, too, yelling obscenities directed at the shooter (who was long gone). I asked him why he was so angry. I told him he should be thanking the Man upstairs.

"Muthafucka shot me—the muthafucka shot me," he cried.

"Yeah, I know, but the muthafucka didn't kill you. You DO know he was trying to, don't you?" I inquired, sharply. He didn't have much to say after I brought this revelation to light. We walked him to the ambulance and put him on the stretcher, much to his disliking, slapped an ice pack on his head, and off we went.

Apparently the shooter's high-quality firearm either misfired or was too far away to penetrate this guy's hard head.

Sooner or Later You Get Burned

"Medic 16, Medic 16," came the call.

"Medic 16, Charles and Centre, in service," I responded.

"Medic 16 respond, Brookfield and Whitelock for a shooting," came the voice. This fine neighborhood, called Reservoir Hill, was in our first due area. The neighborhood entertainment revolved around a liquor store located at the intersection where we were heading (in case you remember this intersection being mentioned before and thought I was running out of ideas). Bonnie and I arrived to find a man who appeared to be in his thirties, leaning against a police car, in handcuffs. The cops told us he was under arrest for attempted murder. His twenty-two automatic misfired and blew up in his hand.

We wrapped his hand up and had the cops handcuff him again before we loaded him into the ambulance. They would follow us to the hospital unless the perp was considered dangerous, an escape threat, or freaking out, then they would ride in the back of the ambulance, and they hated that. I carried a "Black Widow," stainless steel boot dagger, inside my right boot all the time, even on day work. Having kooks like this one on board didn't really bother me.

The calls you just read about were few. The majority of the shootings I handled were worse. By majority I mean, the stories you just read are ones that didn't really kill someone on the spot. We usually didn't haul the dead ones. We'd get to the call, look at the mess and say "Yep, they're dead," then be on our way. Baltimore city medics were the only medics in the state that had that power. By the time the police investigation was through, the Medical Examiner was waiting to haul them to the city morgue. There were enough of these calls to write a few chapters on but they would be very repetitious and basically talk of brains, blood, guts, big holes where vital organs were located, blood running down the street, and so on. I'll spare you the details.

I was detailed to Medic 7 one night trick. *The night trick from hell. Actually it was the night trick IN HELL.* World famous, Medic 7 was the busiest medic unit in the nation. It was a Saturday night in August, the night before a full moon, at the beginning of the month. The temperature was eighty-four at eleven at night and the humidity was "Baltimore-style" (I had a wet towel around my neck the whole night). It was all the ingredients for a royal ass-whipping and that's exactly what I got.

In the short time that I was in the station before the drudging, I noticed that the medics here had the nicest bunkroom I'd ever seen. The bunks were all perfectly made—it was nice and dusted, with a big TV. It looked like a freakin' model firehouse bunkroom. I found out why, the hard way. They were never there, *ever!* We had to come back from the hospital "out-of-service" at the end of the shift so we could go home and I had three more nights of this abuse to go.

A Different Kind of Family

Medic 7 was a true "East Side" medic unit. It's first due area was right in the middle of what we called "Deepest, Darkest" with lots of low-income housing projects. It truly was a "war wagon." The back of the ambulance smelled like something I couldn't identify, it was less than sanitary, poorly stocked, and it ran like hell. I just hoped that it would make it through the night. Hell, I hoped I would make it through the night.

"Medic 7, Medic 7," the radio blared.

"Medic 7, Gay and Monument Streets, in service," I replied.

"Medic 7 respond, 5957 Monument Street, for a stabbing," was the call. We were about fifteen blocks away. No engine company was going with us, which was unusual and usually meant we'd need one. Murphy's Law was sure to apply again. Sure enough, we roll up to find the cops on the sidewalk out front, doing CPR on this kid that looked to be in his teens.

"MEDIC 7 TO COMMUNICATIONS, ENGINE COMPANY PRIORITY 1 FOR A FULL ARREST," I requested, as we pulled in front of the address.

"OK Medic 7, Engine 51 is being dispatched," was the return. This kid had a stab wound to his left upper chest, right over his heart. This was not good, and the cop that was doing CPR said that the kid's older brother (who was in custody) had stabbed him.

"He took my crab," the cop said.

"What?" I said back.

"His brother said he stabbed him because 'He took my muthafuckin' crab,'" the cop whispered. The boys had gotten a dozen crabs this evening and, apparently, Junior took the biggest one that his older brother had staked a claim to. So big brother stood up and stabbed little brother in the chest with a butter knife. His own sibling was DRT (dead right there—that's where the term 'dirt nap' comes from). We worked on the kid and after doing everything we could, beat feet to Hopkins Trauma. It was a futile effort and we knew it would be. Too many times we go through the motions, knowing what the outcome is going to be. I admit, miracles do happen and we'll give it our best shot every time, but there would be no miracle tonight.

You Can't Ever Get Lazy…Ever

One of the biggest things that bugged me about my job was working with lazy people. My parents were the greatest. They gave me all the tools that I needed to survive in the "real" world. They taught me how to cook, sew, do laundry, iron my clothes. They taught good hygiene and the "whole ten yards." (A chief of mine used to say that all the time and it finally made sense. Nine yards is one short of a first down.) They also taught me that if you're gonna do a job, do it right the first time and do the whole job. Half-assed didn't cut it in my house.

As a paramedic, you have to do the job right and do the whole job. Unlike the weatherman (who gets paid really good money to guess what the weather's gonna be), a medic can make no mistakes. If you make mistakes, people die. If you do a job half-assed, people will die. If you get lazy, people will die.

"Medic 16, Medic 16," came the call.

"Medic 16, North and Howard, in service," Jim replied, as he grabbed the mike before me.

"Medic 16 respond with Engine 32, Broadway and Lombard, sick on the street," was the response.

Jim was detailed with me this shift. We heard Medic 10 go to the same intersection for the same thing about twenty minutes earlier. We figured it was probably a refusal, GOA (gone on arrival), or the infamous "not a medic case."

Another luxury the medics in Baltimore City had was the ability to refuse to take someone to the hospital. No other jurisdiction in the state allowed that but, because there was so much abuse of the services in the city, this was acceptable. I didn't like it. You had better be very sure that the person wasn't actually having a problem before you refused to haul him. Especially with most of them being "liquored" up. Alcohol can mask a lot of illnesses and injuries. You can't assume (make an ass out of you and me) they're just drunk. You'd be setting yourself up for a big fall, as you'll see.

Engine 32 had been on the scene for a few minutes when we arrived. They were hovering around this young guy who was sitting on the sidewalk, leaning against a building with his legs straight out and crossed. He looked pretty comfortable, actually. I walked up to the captain from Engine 32.

"He's drunk. We were just here with 10," he said.

"I know, I heard," I replied. I proceeded to roust this guy up and hopefully get him moving. If he gets moving, he'll eventually sober up or walk to the next medic unit's territory and they can deal with him. Don't laugh, I had a call for the same drunk three times in an hour, one shift. He'd walk three blocks and pass out, walk three blocks, and pass out. Every time he passed out in front of a different place, someone would call 911. I finally went nose-to-nose with the cops and got them to take him in (or take him somewhere out of my first due because I was tired of seeing his drunken ass—I didn't care). Sooner or later he'd fall and get hurt or get hit by a car, then I'd have to take him anyway.

Meanwhile, back at the ranch, Jim and I tried to help this guy to his feet. I was on his right side, and Jim on his left. As I put my hand under his armpit, he doubled over in pain. We sat him back down, pronto. Something was up. Even though it was seventy-five degrees out, I had to remove his quilted flannel shirt. Street people usually wear everything they own, regardless of the season. As I removed his right arm from the shirt I found the source of the pain. It was a small caliber gunshot wound, about eight inches below his armpit. This was not a good thing.

Engine 32 had called Communications earlier requesting the police and told them it was the same patient that they had with Medic 10. Somebody was in deep shit and it wasn't us. You can't just walk up to a drunk, nudge him a couple times, and leave, calling him "not a medic case." I didn't want to be that medic from 10. That was a big-league mistake. I didn't feel sorry for him though. I was just as tired as he was. You can never let fatigue affect your performance, ever. If you think it might, you better go home. It's safer for everyone. We got this guy packaged up and hauled him to Hopkins Trauma. He had good lung sounds on the affected side the whole time. He may have been another lucky one. I wasn't lucky on this night—I just did my job.

Chapter 7
Welcome to the World

One thing about my job became very tiring, very quickly. It wasn't the long night tricks, endless paperwork, accountability, or hauling the same dumb asses over and over again, it was *death*.

Seeing people die or getting killed was *very* tiring. A lot of it was senseless disregard for human life. A lot of it was just life itself and the realization of how short life can be for some people. To finally be able to bring a life into this world was a beautiful and uplifting experience.

Really Sick

One thing that irritated the firefighters in the department was being detailed to another station. We are all creatures of habit but it seemed that this act just made them unbearable. Unless, of course, they were detailed to a station that had fewer runs than theirs. Then it was vacation time and they were more worthless. The only thing worse was being detailed, and the person they were detailed in for was detailed to the medic unit—the "double whammy." Sorry about your luck.

Mick was detailed from Engine 13 to Engine 1 for Jim, one night. Jim was detailed to the medic unit with me but called in sick, so Mick was my man. Word had it, he was a bit of a looney toon. Of course, anyone in this business has to be a little whacky. The saying was "You must be crazy to run into a burning building when the rats are running out"—not a bad point. Mick was a Viet Nam vet and very likable. He had just gotten the double whammy and didn't seem to care. I liked his attitude. As the night went on, we got to know each other a little better and I can understand why people would think he wasn't playing with a full deck. We both knew that we had a job to do and would make the best of it.

"Medic 16, Medic 16," the call came.

"Medic 16, Saint Paul and Twenty-Ninth, in service," I moaned.

"Medic 16 respond, 1207 Gold Street, second floor, for a sick case," the voice said. Another sicky. Sick cases were general. If the 911 operator wasn't sure what the call was, the caller was so drunk they couldn't understand them, or it sounded like a "shit call" (one that really wasn't an emergency) it was classified as a "sick case."

Mick and I arrived at the residence. It was an old, three-story row home with two or three apartments, which describes most of the homes in our first due area. I grabbed my aid bag and we climbed the dark stairwell to the second floor. I knocked and shouted, "Fire Department!" No answer. I cracked the door open and hollered again, "Fire Department!" Don't ever open the door and walk in. You may be greeted with four legs and teeth, or worse. I can't tell you the number of times I knocked on the wrong door or we were given the wrong address.

We heard a moaning voice, "I'm in here." We entered and there, on the couch, was a teenage-looking girl with her pants down to her knees, lying on her side, about to give birth. The baby's head was crowning, but not completely out yet. Sick case my ass—*Shit.* I had never done this before and neither had Mick.

"Go get the OB kit and step on it, bro," I ordered. Mick hit the door and all of a sudden it sounded like he fell down the steps. I ran to the door and looked. He was already on his way back up the stairs with the kit, and what a relief to know he wasn't lying in a crumpled heap at the bottom of the steps.

We returned to matters at hand and, after a quick interview of the patient, learned that this was her fourth child. Even though her contractions were thirty seconds apart I kept saying, "Not yet, don't push yet, God damn it." It was her fourth child and she looked like she was fifteen, for Christ's sake. She was actually eighteen and the thought of four children at such an early age made my head spin. She was ready to deliver. Mick and I got a sterile sheet under her and another for after the delivery. My heart was jumping out of my chest. I knew that once I got her on her back with her legs flexed (the delivery position) that it would probably be quick. Boy, was I right. I got ready for the next contraction, with my hands close to her to support the baby's head when it delivered. Here comes the contraction and, POW…baby. I had just experienced what I had only read about in the past—an explosive delivery. I caught that baby like a freakin' screen pass. I had gooey crap all over my arms and shirt but at least it wasn't a "bouncing baby." I put the baby down on the fresh sheet and immediately suctioned, mouth first, then nose. A little whack on the bottom of the feet and, presto, we have ignition. That was the greatest cry I had ever heard. It was a little girl and she was not a happy camper. The rest of us were.

"Medic 16 to Communications, give me a time for childbirth," I called.

"2130, Medic 16," was the reply.

"Sixteen copied, 2130 hours. Give us an Engine Company, Priority 3 for assistance," I acknowledged.

"OK, Medic 16, Engine 25 en route," came the voice.

"Good job, brother," Mick said, as he patted me on the back. I felt like the new father. What a wonderful feeling. Am I supposed to feel like this at work? This feels good and I like it. I want to do it again! We cleaned the baby up, clamped and cut the umbilical cord, wrapped her in a blanket, and gave her to Mom. That was the shortest trip to a hospital I ever experienced. I wanted to drive around town just to make this feeling last. Somehow I knew it wouldn't.

They Almost Made It

Living in the Mid-Atlantic region of the country is pretty nice. You get to experience all four seasons. Over the years I grew to dislike winter, snow, ice, cold, and wind. Hell, I'm a warm weather person. I found it much easier to cool off when it was hot than warm up when it was cold. I didn't like working in it either, slipping and sliding all over the place. It was especially fun when you're trying to carry a patient or stretcher.

I believe that snow, or just the forecast of snow, has a strange effect on people. The universal reaction is to run to the store and buy milk, bread, and shit paper. What's that all about? (especially the shit paper part) Snow definitely has an effect on pregnant women. I guess it's the fear of being stranded and going into labor that induces labor. It just seemed like whenever it snowed, you heard a story about some woman giving birth somewhere other than where she should have. We were in quarters one night during a hellacious snowstorm. It was falling at a rate of an inch an hour and we had at least a foot on the street.

"GONG."

"Medic 16 respond, North and Eutaw, for a maternity in the blue minivan." the voice echoed. At least we were close. This call was only two blocks up the street. I looked out the door and saw the van with its four-way flashers on at the intersection. Our ambulance was equipped with four-wheel-drive so it was no problem getting there.

David and I arrived and walked up to the van. After delivering a few babies you get the feel of it and you know when it's time to go or time to stay. This one was staying. Her contractions were close and we figured it was better to put the dad and the kids in the back of the ambulance so we had room to work in the van, and had no distractions. Mom was lying on the back seat. We moved the front seats forward and got set up. This was probably my third or fourth delivery and I felt comfortable. The mother had prenatal care and was within a week of her delivery date, so all systems were go. We explained to her that it was safer for all if we delivered it in the van. At this point, I don't think she cared whether we were in the van or in the middle of the street. It was a normal delivery about ten minutes later. We loaded the whole family in the ambulance and David moved the van to the curb. There was no sense in Dad having an accident on the way to the hospital or getting stuck somewhere.

It all seemed so routine to me now. That wonderful feeling I had after my first delivery was just a little more than a good feeling now. I thought to myself, *Am I losing something here?* I had heard the word "calloused" a few times, when people would ask me what I did for a living.

"Oh, you must be calloused, seeing what you see," they'd say.

I didn't like it. *I was exactly the opposite of that,* I thought. I had a drive to help people in need, to help grieving family members, or anyone in a time of crisis. I had a heart and feelings. Inside this hard shell was a softness. I felt a need to find out about myself. My conclusion didn't take long to figure out.

When I was a volunteer and studying to become a CRT, I was invited to sit in with a paid man I had met who was studying for his EMT-P certification. His name was Marty but more affectionately known as Cuz. My brother was a volunteer in Anne Arundel County, too, and had introduced me to Cuz at a party one night. Cuz lived about a half mile from me, and we had become friends. He was a "former" Marine (never ex) and had worked for the county fire department for ten years. He was one of the first CRT's in the state and was very smart—more importantly, "street smart." Cuz became my mentor. I would sit in with him and a few other career paramedics during their study sessions. My God, I felt like the luckiest man on Earth. Not only was I invited to study with this elite group of guys but they actually liked me. The rivalry between the volunteers and career, union firefighters was fierce, even physical at times. Here I was, sitting in the middle of a group that most of my volunteer buddies would have called the enemy. It was a great honor for me and I became eager to be the best, just like them.

The studying paid off. We all completed our missions. Thanks to Cuz, I was able to assess what was going on with my feelings. If I ever had a problem, I'd call him. He was like my personal trainer. He taught me how to deal with life and death without driving myself crazy. Many people that choose the Emergency Services as a career don't have this luxury. It's usually trial and error with their emotions. I had learned earlier from Louie (my first mentor) that you have to learn to deal with your emotions first, before you can deal with someone else's. Cuz took it to the next level. Over the course of my career, I'd see what "burn-out" really was and work hard not to fall victim to it. No easy task, especially for a person with feelings. Was I starting to fall? I called Cuz.

Cuz was always eager to help me. He is the wisest person I have ever met. He put things in perspective for me. I will never forget this analogy.

"Cuz [oh yeah, we called each other Cuz] callused is not the word, programmed, is the word—like a machine programmed to do a job. You know what has to be done and you do it. You do the best you can with the tools you have, like a tradesman. If you don't acquire the desired outcome, you look back and think about what you did. As long as you follow your protocols, perform your skills, and give it your best shot, that's the best you can do. Murphy (Murphy's Law) will always be looking over your shoulder. You have to deal with him, too. Remember that Rule Number 1 is, people die. Rule Number 2 is that you can't change Rule Number 1. Second-guessing yourself or what-if-ing yourself will drive you crazy, quick. Don't lose confidence in your ability to be a good medic because you are a good medic, and don't get emotionally involved. Work like that machine," he said.

This analogy helped me make it through over twenty years in the service. Of course, there were going to be calls that hurt, events close to home that hurt, and pain thrown at me from every angle. Cuz's phone rang at least once a week and he always knew the answer. He is retired and living in Florida and to this day, my most respected friend. I was still a relatively young man with a long road ahead of me. I would learn that every day is an experience and there should be a lesson learned every day. One thing I learned quickly was don't "go it alone." Don't try to be a hero or a macho tough guy. It's a hard fall. Don't be afraid to seek help or advice from people. I met a lot of people over the course of my career that helped me make it down the road. I never would have met them if I hadn't asked for their help, advice, or opinions. It wasn't a road I wanted to travel alone, and if anything, it made me more of a man.

Chapter 8
What's Wrong with This Picture?

I can attest to one thing, this occupation will make a *"worldly"* person out of you and it doesn't take long. I used to think that going to the horse races was similar. To me, the racetrack was like a miniature world. All races, all income levels, all intermingled in one place, at one time, with one goal. It was cool. Well, the same can be said for this job. When people would ask me about my job I would say (loudly, with a few beers in me), *"I'm a street doctor practicing gutter medicine. I've seen them beaten up, burnt up, cut up, and shot up— run over by cars, trucks, buses, and trains. Have I seen it all? Ha! That'll never happen! I take care of the homeless troll that lives under the expressway, the millionaire lawyer that lives in Bolton Hill, and everyone in between. I'm a fuckin' street medic."* After that spiel, they'd quietly move away from me. Too bad no truer words can describe it. Speaking of trolls... *"WTF was that?"*

It was my second month at Medic 16 when I became a friend with another firefighter from Engine 1. His name was Doug. I had learned that Doug lived in the county, close to me. I actually drove past his house on the way to work. One night, I was sitting in the back of the engine room, watching TV. The medics, usually, would never make it to the second floor before picking up another call, so we had a table and chairs, and a TV in the back of the station, behind the parked equipment. Now that I think about it, there were times when I slept in the front seat of the ambo, when we backed into the station, too tired to even get out.

There was a soda machine, too, that had quite a history. Stories were told about the blank button on the soda machine. There was one for Coke, Root Beer, 7UP, Orange Crush, and a blank. You could put your quarter in and the blank would serve you a nice, cold Budweiser. Times had definitely changed and the chances of that happening today were remote. A soda for a quarter?

That must have been a while ago.

There was a metal door that led to the street behind the firehouse. The door was supposed to stay locked at all times (to keep the riff-raff from wandering in). Doug had shown me pockmarks in the bricks on the back of the building. It seems there was a shootout there one night. The building was old and was located right next to the Jones Falls Expressway (the main highway into the city from the north). The entrance ramp to the expressway was right next to the station and you could actually see traffic on the expressway from the lieutenant's office on the second floor.

There was a rare lull in the action on this particular evening and I actually got to sit down and watch a little TV. Doug was at the watch desk located in the front of the station. He had a small TV in there and was required to stay on "watch" for four hours. It was a time-honored tradition of the department that wouldn't go away, even though we had a modern alert and radio system. I guess they figured that if someone banged on the door for help and everyone was upstairs, no one would hear them, or that they weren't smart enough to pick up the phone in the alarm box mounted on the front of the building. In any case, I was happy to be sitting still.

I got pretty involved in the baseball game I was watching. The "night lights" were on up front, so aside from the TV and the soda machine, it was fairly dark where I sat. All of a sudden the back door opened and this huge, dark figure entered the building. It was carrying a large glass jar. I got up out of my seat and bolted to the watch desk.

"Doug, something just came in the back door," I frantically whispered as I clutched his vest with a death-like grip.

"What?" he calmly replied. I was freaking out.

"There's a fuckin' monster or something back there," I gasped. I was trying to whisper and scream at the same time. I thought I was gonna pop a blood vessel in my head. Doug got up, pulled out his Buck knife and opened it as we sneaked along side the engine towards the back. I tried to hide behind him. We could hear water running in the wash basin. I fumbled for my boot knife and stopped, as Doug peeked around the back of the engine.

"You fuckin' goof, that's just the Troll," he blared out, as the huge thing turned to look at us.

I quickly walked to the front and Doug followed. He was laughing so hard I thought he was going to piss himself. Troll? What's the Troll? He told me the

Troll was a homeless man that lived under the expressway, across the ramp next to the firehouse. He would frequent the wash basin for his fresh water supply. He stood well over six feet tall and wore a long black raincoat, black shoes, and a black knit hat that hardly contained the biggest afro hair I had ever seen. It had to be a foot high. As soon as I heard him leave, I made Doug go back and lock the door. I wasn't going back there. I was actually happy to get my next call.

Wheat, Not Rice

"Hey, you guys are getting a run," Doug chirped. He hit the gong once. The signals from the watch desk were once for medics, twice for the engine, three times for the truck, and ring the hell out of it if we were dumping the house (meaning everyone was going). There was a button on the watch desk that rang this huge brass gong that you could hear across the street. The printer would spit out the call just before the audible radio alert. That's how Doug knew we had a run.

"Medic 16 respond in the rear of number 801 West North Avenue, for an assault. Police on the scene," the voice called. Bonnie slid down the pole and out the door we went. We were only about five blocks away from this one. We rolled into the alley behind the residence. I hated alleys. They were dark, normally cluttered with trash (real and human) or illegally parked cars. People that didn't want to walk the street, namely drug dealers and their customers, prostitutes and their customers, or anyone up to no good, frequented them. We always turned the emergency lights off and turned all the floodlights on so we had a half-assed idea what or who was where.

On this night, the police were tending to a middle-aged female that had been beaten about the face. She was a mess. Both eyes were swollen, her lips were both fat and bleeding, and her nose was the same. Someone had flogged the hell out her. The police had finished their report and we walked her to the ambulance. I did the best I could to comfort her, emotionally. I felt bad for her, regardless of why she had received this treatment, especially from a man, if that's what a woman-beater thinks they are. Two things I could not (and still can't) tolerate were woman-beaters and child-beaters. These are not men (or women in some cases). These are cowards. I'm getting pissed just thinking about them. It took a lot of restraint to keep my mouth shut and my fists at my sides when dealing with them.

I took a moist, sterile dressing and cleaned my patient up, then I wrapped an ice pack in gauze and laid it across her nose and eyes. She was sobbing. The hospital was about five minutes away. We arrived and she was quickly transferred to the care of the ER. One of the biggest pains about my job is the paperwork. We had to fill out a "DOT sheet," for the state records, which looked like an SAT answer sheet, then write a narrative report describing the call, mechanism of injury, extent of injury, and care given. It was very time-consuming but necessary from the legal aspect. If I was going to be called as a witness in a criminal or civil case, I'd want a decent recollection of what, where, and when. It happened pretty often.

I sat in the EMS Room at the hospital (Provident—we called it *Jungle General*) filling out my paperwork. A few minutes had passed when the charge nurse walked in. She was a rotund, black woman named Wanda. She was personable every time I had ever dealt with her and I liked her a lot. We would joke around and I loved to make her laugh, when we weren't working together seriously.

"Uh-huh, I see what y'all is bringin' me tonight," she barked.

"Whatcha talkin' 'bout girlfriend?" I rattled back.

"Uh-huh, that woman you just brought in, well, you should've taken a betta look, lova," she scorned.

"NO!" I said with my mouth gaping.

"Uh-huh, she look like that cuz somebody got wheat when they thought they was gettin' rice," she said, just before we both broke out in gut-busting laughter.

No shit. Maybe if her, or his, or its...face was less swollen it would have been a little more obvious but I had no clue that she was a he. Proof again that Medic 16 had the strangest clientele of any city unit. I had been detailed to most of the other units and never saw anything comparable to good old 16.

Doing My Part

Jim and I had become pretty close away from the job, as I mentioned earlier. One shift, he told me that the firefighters from the Burn Center Fund were having a "bar night" at Bullwinkle's on Eastern Avenue. He asked me to come have a couple beers for a good cause. It was the last day of day work so I agreed, since we were off the next day. It was a $5 cover, $1 drafts, and drink specials to raise money for the Fund.

Nine years ago, the city firefighters got together and started the Firefighter's Burn Center Fund to benefit the Baltimore Regional Burn Center. A lot of firefighters had gone there for treatment, as you can imagine, and this was a way of saying thanks for the great care that they received.

Jim was on the board of directors for the firefighters. They raised a nice chunk of change every year. They wouldn't purchase things for the Center that just benefitted firefighters. They would buy TV's, VCR's and tapes, books, toys, and the like, for the children's ward at the Center, too. When I heard that, I immediately wanted to join the cause.

I arrived at the bar and met Jim. Later that evening he introduced me to Todd from Engine 5 and Dale from Engine 50. They were on the Fund's board, too. In the months that followed, the four of us became a tightknit group. I went to every bar night and function that I could. We would meet after the Fund's monthly meeting or after the monthly union meetings and hop the local "titty bars." We referred to it as "slummin'."

The camaraderie of the city firefighters far outweighed that of the county. The city department had over 1,900 workers at the time. It was the biggest "family" I had ever been a member of. I was happy that I was able to fit in.

Oooo…Oooo…That Smell

One night, after a union meeting, Jim and I went slummin'. Todd and Dale had to get home and declined the temptation. Jim and I decided to start out at the Red House. It was a sleazy little joint on the east side of town. We met outside and strolled in like we owned the place.

You know you're slummin' when you walk into a strip joint, the first thing you smell is body odor, and the girl dancing is half-naked with the hood up on the juke box because it quit playing. Jim and I stopped halfway down the bar, looked at each other, and started laughing.

"It doesn't get any better than this, brother," he shouted. The place was pretty crowded and fairly noisy. I grabbed a bar table while Jim went to the bar to order. That was quicker than waiting for the waitress, who was at the pool table bullshitting with her friends. Jim slid the beers on the table and joined me. We were just relaxing and talking fire department stuff when this young, slender guy walked past us, headed for the back of the bar. I got a whiff of him as he breezed past. Whew. I cringed.

"What's wrong?" Jim asked.

"Whew, the guy that just walked by smelled like a fag," I replied.

"Get outta here, you can tell by smellin' him? No way," Jim shouted.

"I'm tellin' ya' bro, I can tell. I've been at 16 long enough. Trust me on this one, I can tell," I returned.

"Ah bullshit. I don't believe you," Jim countered.

"OK man, whatever," I said. Just then, the guy came out of the bathroom and walked toward us. Jim had his back to him so he didn't know. As he passed us I just cringed again and a cold chill went down my spine. Jim shook his head. The waitress, who wasn't far behind the guy, saw me cringe and walked up to me. She grabbed my arm.

"Ewww, I know," she said, and gave us the little, "gay wave" thing with her hand as she walked away.

"NO SHIT. You could tell! How could you tell?" Jim blasted.

"I told ya', man. I can just tell. I've smelled that odor too many times, bro," I gloated. Maybe it's just a sense that I could only acquire from 16. Let me try to explain what I detect and why. I'm really not sure but this is my best medical guess. It sounds gross but I think that when a male ingests semen (or in a lot of cases has it injected), it gives him a distinct body odor. It smells like ammonia (like broccoli, cabbage, or asparagus make your piss stink and give you a stronger body odor). Hey, that's my best shot. One of my old girlfriends used to cut hair. Now and then, we would give her shampoo boy a ride to, or from, work. She would talk about his alternate behavior, so I knew that he was flaming, for sure. He had that smell. I finally told her that we were done playing "fag taxi" because it took me two hours to get the smell out of my car every trip.

Wasting Time

As you might imagine, not every call we responded to was a "true" emergency. Truthfully, half of them weren't. Some were legitimate calls or what were referred to as "good intent" calls. As the number of cell phones increased, so too did the number of "good intent" calls. Everyone wants to be a hero but, please, please, please verify the incident before you call 911. Hot things steam, especially in cold weather. Numerous times units will respond to building fires just to find a steaming dryer vent or reports of car fires that were just overheating.

A lot of calls were obviously abuse of the system. It, too, got worse and worse as years progressed. Using the ambulance as a taxi was a common occurrence. We once took a sick case to "Jungle General," just to have him get off the stretcher and bolt out the back door of the ambulance as we arrived at the ER. A mall was right across the road.

One night we were about to clear Sinai Hospital, in the Pimlico section of town, after taking a patient there. I was driving on this particular night and David was riding aid (which means he would ride in the back with the patient). As we started to pull away from the ER, I looked in the rear view mirror and saw something move in the back of the ambulance. I slammed on the brakes, threw the shifter in park, and shot out the door. I got to the back of the ambulance and opened the back doors. Sure enough, we picked up a passenger while we were inside finishing up paperwork.

"Get the fuck out of my ambulance," I hollered at the top of my lungs. David got out and joined me as the middle-aged man climbed out and headed for Northern Parkway.

"…and tell your friends, this ain't no taxi, dumb ass," I added as he walked away. David cracked up.

This guy had no idea where we were going but he was going with us. Some people don't care about you or anyone else for that matter. They'll call 911 for a ride and could care less if you have to wait for a medic unit to come across town when you're having the "big one" and seconds count, let alone minutes. There's a law against it but most people know all the right words to use to get themselves a free ride.

A True Emergency

Doug was detailed to the ambulance on occasion. He was another firefighter who didn't mind the abuse of the medic unit as long as he was working with me. We had become pretty good friends away from the station, too. After we realized we were neighbors, we started carpooling. He owned a 1952 Chevy Suburban painted primer red. It ran. That's all I can say about it. He enjoyed the modern day amenities of my Dodge Shelby Charger and all the creature comforts like heat and air conditioning. I always drove, needless to say.

"Medic 16, Medic 16," the radio blared.

"Medic 16, Calvert and Thirty-Third, in service," I shouted back.

"Medic 16 respond, number 2716 Saint Paul Street, for a sick case on the third floor," came the call. Doug and I rolled up in front of the three-story rowhome. A lot of Hopkins and Art Institute students lived in this area. The homes weren't too bad in this block. Most had been renovated and rented out by the owners. We made the climb in a lit stairwell, for once.

"Fire Department!" I announced as I knocked. A college-aged male, who had a large bandage over his right ear, greeted us. We followed him into the apartment. I didn't get a response when I asked him what the problem was, at the front door. He just turned and walked into the place and sat down in a large, ratty-looking overstuffed chair.

"Can you change my bandage, please?" he asked, in a voice that automatically stereotyped him. He was rubbing his crotch with one hand and sitting on the other.

"Excuse me? You called 911 to have an Advanced Life Support Medic Unit, that happens to be at a premium these days, respond here to change your fucking bandage?" I asked, in a loud amazed tone.

"Come on, Doug, we're outta here," I barked as I headed for the door. This guy had a cyst lanced on his earlobe and a drain inserted and was more interested in two men in uniform in his apartment than his bandage.

"Medic 16 to Communications, in service, not a medic case," (echoing in the stairwell) I called.

"OK, 16, in service at 2055." As we got back to street level, Doug said, "Hey. bro, I think that guy liked you."

"Fuck off, I think he liked US, you ass. You do look manly in your uniform, you know," I fired back. We laughed together as readied ourselves for the next true emergency.

41-30

Doug and I would, inevitably, end up at O'Brien's Pub on the way home in the mornings. It was our favorite "watering hole" on our days off. After sucking down coffee all night to stay awake during night tricks, a few cold beers in the morning was enough to let us get a couple hours of sleep during the day (so we could get up and start the cycle all over again). Henry was the owner of this small Irish bar that featured ice-cold draft beer and frosted mugs.

Henry and I would go to the horse races together quite often. I was one of his favorite customers. Doug and I would arrive around seven-thirty in the morning (in uniform) and knock on the plate glass window in the front of the bar. Henry would get up from his coffee and daily racing form and let us in. Doug used to refer to this as 41-30 time. We would carve the numbers 41-30 in our frost-covered mugs with our fingernails. Article 41, Section 30 of the Fire Department Rules and Regulations clearly defined "Actions detrimental to the good name of the Department." Sitting at a bar and drinking beer in uniform would qualify as one of them. We didn't care. Night work sucked. We were all wired out on caffeine and both needed to sleep.

If I had to describe Doug to you, it would sound like this. He's in his early thirties, stands about six-three, and weighs all of 150 pounds. He always wore his fire department baseball hat at work and loved the great outdoors. He was a weapons aficionado and a soldier of fortune mercenary in his previous life. I'm totally convinced. (Hell, he subscribed to the magazine *Soldier of Fortune*). He had handguns, rifles, shotguns, black powder rifles, knives, machetes, and swords. I actually watched him build an ocean kayak in his garage from a set of plans from *Popular Mechanic* magazine. The guy was amazing. He took me camping a couple times, too—they were a trip each time.

The first time we went camping was bad. We went back country, Skyline Drive, Virginia. It was thirty-two miles south of Luray, Virginia, with no shelter other than the two-man tent we carried. No campfires were allowed unless we needed it to survive the cold and a small, one-burner, propane-fueled stove fit neatly in my pack. We were going for two days. Doug's pack weighed fifty-five pounds and mine was forty-five. It was April and we took his truck because we couldn't fit all the gear in my car and we didn't think we'd need a heater. He parked the truck in an empty parking lot just past mile marker thirty-two. We got our packs on, locked the truck, placed our itinerary in a zip lock baggie under the windshield wiper (in case we were eaten by a fucking bear, I guessed) and headed for the trail. I stopped at the trail entrance and looked at what was ahead.

It was downhill, and I mean downhill. It looked to me like straight down. *We're going down there?* It was 1,500 feet of steep, rocky, winding-assed trail, right from the start. I had to stop every two or three minutes because I was getting shin splints, for God's sake. I never thought going downhill would be tough. It took, what seemed like hours.

We really had to struggle not to get moving too fast, especially with the weight we were carrying. By the time we got to the bottom we needed a long break but it was worth the effort and pain. It was very serene and I knew why

Doug loved coming here. It was an escape from the world we lived and worked in. I loved this place, too. All I could hear were birds chirping and the rustle of wind through the leaves. I couldn't recall the last time I had heard that sound.

We ventured along the trail which was in a valley now, and was fairly level. We never heard another voice, traffic, horns honking or, most importantly, a siren or a gong. It was nearly paradise. I would stop now and then, to take a deep breath, listen, and smell the serenity. All of the sudden, out of nowhere, whoooooosssshhh! Whoooooosssshhh! We both hit the dirt. Two military fighter jets flying at treetop level zoomed by. They, obviously, like to come through the valley on maneuvers. That scared the hell out of us. We just lay there for a couple minutes before getting up and dusting ourselves off. There's no warning when a 500-mph jet approaches. Gooooooo...Navy!

We found a line of pine trees along a stacked stone wall that had been built during the Civil War. The sun was setting and we set up camp before it got dark. I don't know about Doug, but I was out cold in record time. Unfortunately, our sleep was short-lived. A couple of hours after crashing out, I awoke to find the foot-end of the cocoon tent touching our legs and the sound of sleet hitting the fabric. It was snowing. I nudged Doug and alerted him. We both kicked our legs upward and got the snow to fall off the tent then dozed off. In what seemed like minutes, we had to repeat the motions. It was really snowing hard. This time, we didn't doze off. I was getting anxious. My breathing was fast, my heart was racing, and I had broken out in a sweat. I thought I was having a panic attack but didn't want Doug to think I was a lightweight, so I kept quiet. I knew he was awake and noticed that he was breathing fast, too. Finally I announced, "Man, I wish I could get back to sleep. I'm having a little trouble breathing."

"Yeah, me too." Doug replied, as he flipped his flashlight on. We looked at each other, and the thought must have struck us at the same time. We both flipped over in our sleeping bags and started unzipping the door of the tent. After getting the door opened we had to push about six inches of snow away from the door cover. Suddenly a rush of fresh air hit us. Ah, oxygenated air. Every time we kicked the snow off our feet, snow slid down the front of the tent and covered the air flap. We had been rebreathing the air in the tent for about two hours. The oxygen was gone and we were both hyperventilating. No wonder we were freaking out. Within a couple of minutes, we were both sound asleep again.

We got up the next morning to find seven or eight inches of snow. It had probably stopped right after we cleared our air vent. We packed and were anxious to head for the truck. It was going to be a long day. We had to go six miles and the last quarter mile was straight up. We knew we had to cross the creek that we had waded across yesterday, but when we got to the crossing we noticed the water had risen and it looked impossible to cross. We started bushwhacking along it. Doug took out his machete and started hacking at the brush as I closely followed. I was glad I was with a mercenary. The last thing you want to do when camping in back country in cold weather is get wet. All I could think of was dying of hypothermia. Doug and I had bushwhacked about a half mile when we found a large tree that had fallen across the creek. I thanked God for putting it there for us. The tree was covered with snow and we knew we would both have a wet crotch when we got to the other side. That's one place where you lose a lot of body heat. Out of the blue, I asked Doug to turn around. I took two large black trash bags out of his pack. They were about three feet long.

"Watch me," I said to him. I spread the first bag out on the tree and climbed aboard. I spread the second bag out in front the first, then shimmied on to it. I reached back and got the first bag and repeated the motions. I did this until I was on the other side, as dry as I was when I started. Doug was standing on the other side grinning. I think he liked it. I found a softball-sized rock and dropped it in one bag, then put the other bag inside and slung the works across the creek, making him jump out of the way. He called me a name and followed my lead across the tree without a problem.

Our journey continued toward the great ascent. I was surprised at the amount of ground we had covered when we finally arrived at the trail's ascent. I guess that when you feel the threat of impending death, you walk faster, or something. We started the climb upward. One thing we had noticed was the closer we got to the truck, the more snow we encountered. The climb seemed shorter than the descent. We were at the truck in no time. It had around ten inches of snow on it but was a welcome sight. Doug hopped in and cranked it up as I brushed the ton of snow off of it. We tossed the packs in and headed north.

A ranger had, apparently, gotten our itinerary and left a note for us. We saw it stuck to the windshield after driving a couple of miles. Doug stopped the truck and peeled the frozen baggie from the glass. The note read: "Campers and

Hikers: Severe Weather Warning. Low pressure forming over Shenandoah Valley tonight. Heavy snow possible." A lot of good it did us now. We approached the gate at the entrance to Skyline Drive, in Luray. It was locked. They had locked us in! Doug laid on the horn in anger. We were pissed. As the horn blared and we yelled every obscenity ever heard, a park ranger appeared from nowhere, walking past the noise and turning to look at us. He shook his head, unlocked the gate, and swung it towards us. He must have been following us for miles without us knowing it. The defroster in the truck was broken and the windows were fogged.

As we wheeled through the open gate, Doug and I agreed, we needed a hot meal. We'll stop at the first place we came to—McDonald's. We ate two meals, each—at least it was hot.

Chapter 9
It Is What It Is

My anniversary date with the city arrived on July 18, 1984. I had been on the job for a year now and my probation period was over. I had actually made it to the rank of Paramedic II. It seemed like longer than that to me. A lot had happened to me in my first year here, both physically and mentally. I felt "seasoned" and, in talking to my friends in the county, had seen and done things that many medics hadn't seen or done in ten years there. I still thought about one day working for Anne Arundel County.

I had applied every year for the past three years but hadn't gotten the call. Honestly, I was getting tired of the abuse that came with the city. The shift hours, the pounding number of calls, and the dumb asses I had to deal with on a daily basis, both in and out of the station, were taking a toll on me. I prayed each night that this year might be the year. More money and less work in a semi-humane environment with state-of-the-art toys is hard not to dream about right now, but I carried on.

China White

Along with the "knife and gun club" on weekends, came another treat, overdoses. Most of them came on Fridays. Money in the pockets of drunks and druggies meant problems for every medic unit in town. My first encounter with an unconscious, non-breathing narcotic overdose was a real learning experience for me.

"Medic 16, Medic 16," the call came.

"Medic 16, in service leaving University [Hospital]," Bonnie replied.

"Medic 16 respond with Engine 52, for an overdose, in the alley behind number 1201 West North Avenue. Police on the scene," chirped the voice. We were about ten minutes away. On every call I received, I tried to mentally prepare myself by picturing the type of emergency I was about to be faced with. With so many protocols and procedures to follow, it helped. I would think of a "plan of attack" for as many possible scenarios as the trip would allow.

Bonnie and I arrived at the scene. A firefighter from Engine 52 was performing ventilation on a male that looked to be in his twenties. Cops and firefighters hated doing medical stuff and were always happy to see us arrive. I grabbed the portable oxygen bottle with the "elder valve" (pressure ventilator) attached. I checked the patient to assure he still had a pulse and relieved the firefighter from rescue breathing. My next thought was to put an EOA tube (a plastic tube inserted into the esophagus to prevent vomit from entering the victim's lungs) in this guy. It was standard procedure for most adult non-breathers. I instructed Bonnie to set the tube up for me. She did so and I inserted it, placing the Elder valve on the tube's mask. He now had a secure airway. Bonnie started an IV while I continued respirations and monitored the patient's status.

Whenever confronted with an unconscious patient, for whatever reason, we had treatment protocols, which included the drugs D50 (Dextrose), and Narcan. The Dextrose was, basically, highly concentrated sugar water that would raise a patient's blood sugar level. It was a diabetic's best friend. It wouldn't harm a patient whose blood sugar was normal, so it was pretty harmless to administer, unless the vein it was being pushed through ruptured (blew) and it infiltrated into the surrounding tissue. You had to push D50 slowly and constantly check for a blood return in the IV to assure that the vein was still good. It was so concentrated that if it did enter the surrounding tissue, it would eat the tissue up (cause necrosis), and that was never a good thing.

The Narcan was a narcotic antagonist. It would reverse the effects of any narcotic, rapidly. By rapidly, I mean, seconds after administrating it. Narcan, like D50, would not have any effect on patients that didn't have narcotics on board, so it was safe to use, too. We were pretty sure that this guy had OD'd; after all, the cops had left this guy's needle and syringe sticking in his arm, I guess to avoid getting stuck with it. Bonnie pushed the Narcan first. The first amp (vial) did nothing. We were allowed to push a total of five amps (2 mg.) before we had to consult the hospital for an order for more. Bonnie pushed two more amps. I saw the patient's eyes blink. He was waking up. His eyes opened, so the Narcan had done the trick.

"How ya' doin', yo?" I said. I was ready to remove the tube. It has an inflatable cuff on it that closes off the esophagus and is uncomfortable to a conscious person. You want to get the tube out quickly after the patient regains consciousness. I wasn't quick enough. In a flash, he sat up and ripped the tube out of his throat. That had to hurt. I tried to hold him down but he had the advantage and pushed me backwards as he stood up, proceeded to rip the IV out of his arm, and walked away.

Oh well, I guess he was feeling better. We all stood and watched as he staggered down the alley with blood running down his arm from the open IV site. We shouted at him to stop and he turned around and flipped us the bird. The lessons learned—don't put a tube in a junkie, be ready to wrestle when they wake up (which is true for a diabetic, too), and junkies get pissed off when you push Narcan and ruin their $100 high.

"Medic 16 to Communications," I called.

"Medic 16?"

"We treated the patient and he left the scene. Engine 52 is clearing and we'll be in service after clean up—about five minutes," I advised.

"OK 16, patient left the scene at 1724," the voice acknowledged. We had seven unconscious, non-breathing overdoses in our first due area that night. The one I just told you about was the only one we handled. Of the seven, three never woke up, at all—they died. I thought to myself, either it was some really good shit, or some really bad shit. The outcome was still the same. On the news and in the paper the next day the stories would read, "Toxic doses of heroin, known as 'China White' claimed three lives and sent several others to area hospitals, last night."

I struggled to understand how anyone could inject the unknown into his or her veins in pursuit of the almighty high. A frosty six of Coors Light was all I needed.

It's Eleven PM, Do You Know Where Your Parents Are?

I learned a lot about kids that grew up in the city, too. It was a hard life for them. Growing up without guidance or discipline meant you had to learn lessons the hard way. Sometimes it was tragic and a lot of parents' priorities seemed to be out of order, to me. I was brought up with a belt, stick, or paddle on my ass, and pepper or soap in my mouth. I learned quickly.

David and I were returning from a call on the west side one night and came across a prime example of what I'm talking about. We were sitting at a red light at around eleven on a school night—I think it was a Wednesday or Thursday.

As we patiently sat, a young child (probably eight or ten years old) crossed the street in front of us. He had a small tree branch in his hand and was slapping it on the street as he began to cross. I wondered if his parents knew or even cared that he was out this late. Maybe there was a reason.

As he crossed in front us, he took the branch and slapped it on the hood of the ambulance, never breaking his stride. David yelled at him. He turned around, still walking, flipped us the bird, and continued on his way. As the light turned green, I gave him a blast from the electronic air horn that took a couple years off his life, judging from the way he jumped. He threw the stick at us as we drove away. We just laughed at his pitiful attempt to do us harm. He'll probably be throwing a brick at the next medic unit he sees. I hope it's not us.

Changing Over

Our first line unit was in the shop for maintenance and Doug and I were using a reserve ambulance one shift. The fleet of reserves was less than desirable. When a unit had high mileage and needed replacing, it didn't get sold or salvaged, it became a reserve. The same held true for engines, trucks, and other pieces, too. This particular gem, Reserve Ambulance 29, had a large hole rusted through the floorboard on the passenger's side. If you pulled back the rubber floor covering you could see a stop sign that had been slid under the mat to cover the hole. If you pulled the sign up, you could see the street. You get my point. I was embarrassed to be seen in some of these junkers.

"Changing over," or the moving of equipment from one unit to another, became one of my most dreaded duties. It was more tolerable if we were changing back into our nice, new, first line unit, but changing out to a reserve was a bitch. You never knew what you were in store for.

One night, Jim and I had a problem with the emergency lights on the new first line unit. We were directed by the EMS duty officer to report to the shop and change over. It usually took a couple hours to do this. None of the reserve units had any equipment on them, which meant we moved almost all of our equipment. Medic 16 was one of five medic units designated as "Mini-Rescue" units. That meant that we carried a Hurst tool (the original and infamous Jaws of Life) on board. Medic units that were housed close to major highways all carried one.

Medic 14 covered the upper Jones Falls Expressway that led into the city from the north and Medic 3 covered I-95 to northeast and both harbor tunnels on the east side of town. Medic 9 covered the tunnels and tunnel thruways to the south in both directions. Medic 12 covered the I-70 extension into town from the west, and we covered the Jones Falls Expressway from midtown to downtown. I was a handy item to have but a pain to move into a reserve. They usually didn't have room for it. We used to say, "Five pounds of shit in a two-pound bag," when we were finished.

Jim and I arrived at the shop at around 8:30 that night. It was August so it was warm and just getting dark. We moved at a slow, steady pace and finished a couple hours later. Jim had talked me into slipping into the bar across the street from the shop before we went back in service. We each slugged down a cold draft. It was rare to drink while on duty but we were hot and sweaty and there wasn't any "brass" at the shop at 10:30 at night. We ran back to the unit and headed for the station. As we drove past the Inner Harbor on Pratt Street, I noticed something.

"Do you have the headlights on, bro?" I asked Jim. The streetlights were bright downtown and it was hard to tell.

"Well, let's put it this way, the button's pulled out," he answered. He turned at the next light and stopped the unit. We both got out and walked to the front. Shit, no headlights. Jim opened the hood and I went to the dash. He wiggled wires and I played with the button. Nothing worked. We checked the fuse and it was good.

"Medic 16 to Communications," I moaned.

"Medic 16?"

"We just completed changeover into Reserve Ambulance 27 and are out of service returning to the shop, no headlights," I griped.

"OK 16, we'll let them know," was the response. We were changing over twice in one night. We turned on the hand-operated spotlights mounted on each side of the windshield and focused them on the street in front of us. Hey, it is what it is. Do the best you can with what junk they give ya'. We each had *two* drafts after the second round of changing over. Jim didn't have to do much arm-twisting the second time. We finally made it back to the station at 1:30 in the morning. It was a five-hour pain in the ass.

Up Your Nose

Doug and I were working together one warm summer day. Summer meant the kids were out of school, the city's pools were packed, fire hydrants were opened, and the "Good Humor" ice cream truck was working overtime.

"Medic 16, Medic 16," came the voice over the radio.

"Medic 16, Northern Parkway and Falls Road, in service," I responded.

"Medic 16 respond, 4503 Liberty Heights Avenue, for a child with a nail stuck in his nose," it replied, with laughter heard in the background.

"How do you mentally prepare for this one, Mark?" I asked myself. Doug was just shaking his head. We arrived at the residence to find an eight-year-old sitting on the couch, not appearing to have a concern. After a quick interview with his mom, I took my penlight and looked in the child's right nostril. I couldn't identify the object but it was very shiny—chrome shiny. It didn't look like a nail. I asked the child what it was. He just shrugged his shoulders. Children get embarrassed easily and I think this was the case.

"Don't worry, Shorty, I'll fix you up," I claimed, as I patted him on the shoulder. Regardless of a patient's age, if you can get them to relax and build their confidence up in you, that's half the battle. Mind over matter really works. I'll prove it later on. I pulled my hemostats (clamps) from my belt pouch, assuring the child that I would stop if I caused him the least bit of pain. He agreed and I shined the light in and opened the clamps up as wide as I could. I grasped the object and gently began to remove it—no problem. It came right out. I guess you want to know what it was? It was a bell out of his dog's chew toy, about the size of a raisin. He thanked me as he ran from the room and out the back door. Another life saved.

Get Rich Quick

Like any other big city, Baltimore has buses and a subway. They're owned and operated by the state and if there was an accident involving either, it was normally low-speed impact or due to sudden stops. It seemed like the ambulance-chasing lawyers weren't far behind and dollar signs always flashed in the eyes of the victims. There was a light dusting of snow on the streets on this particular day, when the radio sounded.

"Medic 16, Medic 16."

"Medic 16, in service, Pine and MLK, leaving University (Hospital)," I answered.

"Medic 16, respond with Engine 2 and Medic 5 for a bus accident at Light and Lee Streets. Police on the scene."

We were only a couple blocks away and arrived at the same time the engine did. It was time to nominate candidates for "Best Actor of the Year" and kind of sad that our society had come to this. We were presented with a Metro bus that had gotten bumped in the rear by a small fuel oil delivery truck. The rear of the bus had a dent in the engine cover and the oil truck had a scratch on its bumper. The injuries were overwhelming. All of the fifteen passengers were writhing in pain, I noticed as I boarded the bus, including the driver. That's funny because I got this sudden, shooting pain in my ass at the same time. It was quite a scene.

I had the officer from Engine 2 call for two more medical units and told him to request them, Priority 3, which meant that the injuries were non-urgent or not life-threatening. We advised the injured to remain still and went to work on the driver. It's true, the mechanism for injury was present, but things just didn't add up. After doing this job enough, you know. I quickly interviewed the driver. He denied ever having previous neck problems. We put a cervical collar (neck brace) on him and slid one of our wooden backboards under his butt. One firefighter supported the end while Bonnie and I supported his head and pivoted him onto it. We slid him forward and got him lying down. He was moaning loudly with every little move or touch. It was sickening. He was a terrible actor. No nomination for this guy.

After getting him positioned on the board, we had to strap him to it. We used three, nine-foot nylon straps. If you were standing outside the door of the bus you'd have thought we were torturing the poor bastard. It was pissing me off but I bit my tongue and carried on. The other "victims" were watching intently. Bonnie and I looked at each other and we both knew what the other was thinking. We were trying to be as gentle as possible but to no avail. It was pure agony. After getting the last strap buckled, I gave it a good tug. The driver moaned in pain, louder than he had previously.

The first of sixteen victims was removed. The medics from 5 were standing outside the door of the bus and told us that they would transport the first of the injured. I knew they just wanted to get out of there. After all, Bonnie and I had done all the hard stuff. I returned to do a quick triage of the remaining injured. Triage is the "sorting" of patients during a disaster to determine which victims need medical attention more than others do. It was easy today. I had fifteen slumped down in their seats holding their necks. Take your pick.

"OK, listen up!" I shouted over the moans. There was a method to my madness. "If any of you would like to seek medical attention on your own, you can do so, within twenty-four hours, and still seek legal advice regarding your injuries. If not, the law requires us to put you in a collar and on a board like we did with the driver. Does anyone want to exercise this option?" I announced. What a line of bullshit, and now you know why I gave the driver that extra "tug" on the strap. Guess what? Every poor, moaning soul raised their hand. Medic 1 and 9 had arrived and I instructed them to put their shit away and grab their clipboards, that all fifteen were refusing treatment and transport. I told Medic 9 go back in service, since a quarter of the medic units in the city were present at this "shit call." I should have gotten the "Oscar" for my performance.

It was amazing to see how therapeutic my announcement was because not one neck was hurting after the refusals were signed. It was simply amazing. I should become one of those TV evangelists. We found another interesting fact before we cleared the scene. A Metro Transit cop had emptied the fare box and determined that there should have only been ten victims on the bus. Five of the so-called injured had seized the opportunity and gotten on the bus after the accident happened. Either that, or the driver had allowed five of his "homeboys" on without making them pay. I had heard stories about people climbing through the windows of buses that had been involved in accidents just to get in on the lawsuit money. I think I had just experienced one of them.

Chapter 10
Them Changes

I was twenty-eight years old when Baltimore City hired me and, frankly, after fourteen months on the job, it was getting old fast. Every shift was a pounding. Not only was it affecting my mind but also, poor diet, sleep deprivation, and drinking every day was taking its toll on me physically.

It was time for things to change. I couldn't go on like this. Heartburn and gastric reflux were making me miserable. I went to the doctor and after a complete physical, was diagnosed with gastric hyperacidity. It's the condition one develops just prior to getting an ulcer. The acid eats your stomach lining up and eventually you develop one.

The medical expert's report made me decide to put my transfer in for Medic 9. It was the second slowest unit (if you could call *any* unit in the city slow) in town and located close to the Anne Arundel County border, on the south side. Their first due area was mainly low to lower-middle-class whites and a lot of industry. Most of the city's chemical plants, oil tank farms, and shipyards were located on the south side of town. It would be a nice change of scenery. The paperwork for my transfer went in on my next day shift. Now, the waiting game began.

The Beat Goes On

In 1985, Baltimore's population was about sixty-five percent black. Working at Medic 16 kept me busy, in what most would refer to as the "ghetto," most of the time. There was one area close to us called Hampden. It was a primarily white neighborhood located up Falls Road. Falls Road ran parallel to the expressway and was easy for us to get to as the second due medic. It was Medic 11's first due area and provided some interesting calls for us.

"Medic 16, Medic 16."

"Medic 16 in service, Druid Park Drive and Auchentroly," I replied.

"Medic 16, respond, Falls and 41st Street for an auto accident." Medic 11 was at the Community College of Baltimore taking a continuing education course. Doug and I were told by our off-going shift that they would be there all morning, so we knew we might have to cover for them. No other unit was dispatched with us on this particular call. At the time, dispatches didn't include an engine, truck, or squad on auto accidents if the 911 call taker determined that the accident was a minor one. Nowadays, they're sent automatically.

Forty-First Street ran off of Falls Road, across the expressway to what's known as TV Hill. That's the highest point of elevation in the city and where the big, local television and radio stations are located. You can see the thousand-foot-tall antenna for miles. Traffic was backed up on Falls as we approached the scene. The police were arriving at the same time from the north. As we came to a stop next to the small crowd of onlookers, I noticed that a television van was on the scene. A photographer had his portable television camera shouldered and had filmed our approach. I recognized one of the local newscasters standing next to the accident vehicle with a microphone. It appeared that a Pinto station wagon had driven onto the sidewalk and struck a retaining wall in front of the local corner store. It didn't look like much of an impact, though. There weren't any signs of urgency from anyone as I got my aid bag from the rear of the unit. It all seemed like a big ado about nothing until one of the bystanders ran up to me and shouted, "She's been shot!"

Startled, I picked up my pace as I walked towards the driver's side. Another bystander was supporting the driver's head that appeared to be a female in her thirties. I took control as he backed away and repeated the message I had just gotten a few seconds earlier. She, indeed, had a small-caliber gunshot wound to her left temple and was unresponsive, breathing erratically in short snorts. Doug had already wheeled the stretcher around next to the car. I opened the door, grabbed the victim under her armpits, and dragged her out far enough for Doug to get a grip on her legs. We placed her on the stretcher and headed for the unit, belts, and buckles dragging. We didn't have time for details—she was in dire straits. I called for assistance.

"MEDIC 16 TO COMMUNICATIONS," I called.

"Medic 16?"

"DISPATCH AN ENGINE COMPANY TO THE TV HILL HELIPAD AND START A MED-EVAC," I commanded.

"OK, Medic 16, Engine 21 will be dispatched and we'll get you an ETA on the Trooper. "

"Also, Medic 16, Medic 11 just cleared their detail and are en route to the scene," the voice on the radio advised.

"Medic 16 OK…16 to 11," I inquired.

"Medic 11."

"PRIORITY ONE PATIENT, TRAUMA ARREST IMPENDING," I told them.

"11 copied, ETA 10." We recognized the voice on Medic 11 as that of our friend, Matt. He lived in the county, not far from us, and joined us at the pub a lot. I used to ride his ass for blowing so much money on the video poker game there. Once we loaded the patient, I placed a cervical collar on her and Doug started assisting her respirations with the trusty elder valve. Her pupils were fixed and dilated similar to that of a dead person's—how ironic.

We rarely called for med-evac helicopters in the city because we were normally only minutes away from any of the three trauma centers located within the limits. Today was different though. This victim needed neurotrauma care, which was a specialty of Shock Trauma downtown. It would take us fifteen minutes to drive there and I needed Doug in the back with me, now. Medic 11 was ten minutes away and the ETA for the med-evac was fifteen.

The Maryland State Police provide all med-evac operations for the entire state. There were eleven of them strategically located across the state. They are referred to as "Troopers," after those who fly them. Trooper 1, from Martin State Airport, was on the way. Medic 11 arrived, Matt jumped in the side door, and relieved Doug.

"Gas on it, bro," I said to Doug, as he headed for the front seat. I had an intravenous line running and had the victim on the heart monitor. Her heart rate was dropping. We took off for TV Hill and I hoped and prayed that she would improve, but deep down inside my gut told me different. I was hoping she wouldn't arrest. Blood loss wasn't the issue here—it was the brain injury. I felt pretty helpless, wishing I could magically do something to make things better. I had done all I could. We could hear the sounds of the Trooper idling on the helipad as we came to an abrupt stop. Doug threw the rear doors open. We took the stretcher out and moved our patient's backboard on to the Trooper's specially made one. I gave the flight medic a quick rundown of the scenario and handed him a copy of my stat sheet that had the patient's vital signs, observations, and times on it, as the four of us carried her towards the waiting bird. We didn't know her name so she was just another "Jane Doe." I knew a lot of John and Jane Doe's, it seemed.

Doug, Matt, and I stood close to the side of the medic unit, away from the helicopter, as it took off. We were sweat-soaked and didn't need a coating of dust and debris blown on us. Matt shook our hands and praised us for our efforts—it felt good. He then says, "Hey, guess what? The county hired me. I start fire school next month."

"What? You son-of-a-bitch!" I spurted, as I slapped him on the arm with the back of my hand.

It was true. We were tossing back a few cold ones at the pub one afternoon, about six months ago, when I mentioned to him that I had put my application in with Anne Arundel County. I had suggested that he do the same. He just balked and mumbled something about starting over with a new department after being with the city for five years. I let it go and, now, he gets hired before I do. He was going to Recruit Class 20 and I was tight. I didn't say two words to him as we drove him back to his station. I even made him ride in the back with the mess we had just made.

It took Doug and I about thirty minutes to get the unit back in service. We did our clean-up at Matt's station and he got us replacement supplies from Medic 11's supply cabinet. Engine 21 returned from the landing site. The lieutenant from the engine came up to us and asked if we knew what had happened at the call. We denied knowing anything other than the woman was shot while at the wheel of her car, bumped into the wall and was probably not going to make it. The lieutenant said that they had stopped at the scene on the way back to the station and talked to the police.

It seems that the woman's estranged boyfriend had been following her down Falls Road. He was driving a Ford van and was two cars behind her in traffic. When she caught the light at Forty-First, he got out of the van, walked up to her car, and fired a single shot without as much as a word. He casually walked back to his van and drove off. She was the first in line at the light and her car just drifted across the sidewalk and came to a stop at the corner store— what a way to go. She died about four hours after arriving at Trauma.

How do we know this? Our fireman "buddies" at the station let us know the minute we got back to our station, later that afternoon. Wigs said it was the top story of the day and that we looked like asses. It was all caught on tape by

ion guys that were there ahead of us. The news was coming on again
to see it. I was hoping we didn't get a call because I had to hear and
see .

I've never had to deal with the media before. What could have made us look
bad? Everything went as well as it could have. I did everything by the book (as
usual). The news came on and there we were—Medic 16 approaching the
scene, Mark, and Doug getting out of the ambulance, cut to Mark dragging the
woman out of car. Stop the clip! Wigs, of all people—Mr. I-Hate-the-
Ambulance-and-Everybody-On-It says, "An auto accident and you drag her
out of the car before you put a collar on her?"

I hit the roof. "You asshole!" I shouted. "The woman's got a bullet in her
head, bumps into a wall at five miles per hour and is getting ready to code on
us, and you think she needs a collar? You stick to riding that fucking ladder
truck, Bud, you're clueless," I added with vigor. Under normal circumstances
I would always put a collar on anyone involved in an auto accident, even if they
didn't complain of neck pain. The "mechanism of injury" is there every time.
In the course, Basic Trauma Life Support for Advanced Life Support
Providers, we are taught to "load-and-go" with certain patients that have life-
threatening injuries or are facing impending death. We call it "swoop and
scoop." This woman was a textbook load-and-go patient, and that's exactly
what we did. The "go" part was delayed because we were the only unit on the
scene and had our hands full with no one to drive us. She eventually got a collar,
but when it was time.

The whole thing made me want to go to Medic 9 even more. I'm sure there
would be a Wigs there too, though. Every station has one.

Hampdenites

During my tenure in this place, that seemed more and more like hell every
shift, I never once had a complaint lodged by anyone I came in contact with.
No patient or family member had a beef that wasn't quelled before I left their
house or the scene of their crisis. I took pride in doing that. Black, white, rich,
or poor, everyone got the best care I could give. I'm not saying it was easy but
I was pretty good at it, until one night.

"GONG."

"Medic 16 respond, number 2601 Roland Avenue for trouble breathing."
the voice echoed. It was just before midnight on a Friday and David and I were

having a routine night, with a couple of drunks, overdoses, and an assault. They were mostly shit calls, with nothing too exciting, but that was about to change. We arrived in front of the address to find a male family member puffing on a cigarette, reeking of alcohol, casually stating, "I think he's dead." I hate it when they do that. I grabbed my bag and oxygen and ran to the door as David climbed in the back of the medic unit to get the heart monitor and drug box. As I entered, two females in the kitchen were sobbing and pointed towards a bedroom down the hall, with the light on.

I found a middle-aged man lying on his back on the bed. He was motionless and didn't respond when I shouted at him. I tried to detect a carotid pulse while watching his chest for any signs of breathing. If he had a pulse, it wasn't much and I never saw his chest move. David entered the room and started to hook up the wires to the heart monitor. I called for help.

"MEDIC 16 TO COMMUNICATIONS," I called

"Medic 16?"

"ENGINE COMPANY FOR A FULL ARREST," I ordered.

"OK 16, Engine 21 will be dispatched at 2245," was the response. I got the airway tube set up while David placed the electrodes on the man's chest. I would give him four or five ventilations with the elder valve, then pause a few seconds to get the tube together.

"Medic 16?" came the call.

"GO AHEAD," I said, without removing the portable mike from my epaulette.

"Engine 21 en route."

"OK," I returned.

I was doing three things at once. I had the tube ready and placed my hand behind the patient's head, flexing it forward. I inserted the tube into his mouth and down his throat. I could smell a strong odor of alcohol. All of the sudden his eyes opened wide and he started swinging and screaming.

"Yu shun a bitch, whacha doin' t'me? I'm gonna kill ya, yu shun a bitch! Stick that fring down my froat! I'm gonna kill ya!" he blubbered. I was so startled that I jumped off the bed, backwards, and just stood there with the tube in my hand, watching this old guy try to find me with his lame attempts at swinging.

"Calm, the fuck, down, will ya, Pop? We all thought you were dead!" I shouted at him. I assumed that the women in the house were his wife and daughter. They ran into the room when they heard his verbal attack and restrained him with a drunken show of affection. Both of them hugged him and sobbed with tears of joy. It was the joy that I had, somehow, brought him back to life. Brought him back to life? This guy was so pickled, they thought he was dead. Hey, so did I. He drank so much alcohol that his respirations and pulses were so depressed they couldn't be detected. I'd never seen that before. He sure got me, though, and I'm sure 21 Engine could hear this goof in the background when I called them on the radio to cancel them.

He was so pissed off at me he wouldn't even sign the refusal when we were ready to leave, twenty minutes later. He wanted me out of his house. His wife signed it and we left.

By the Grace of Gawd

I have to laugh because I just realized that writing this and recalling the stories is kind of like telling jokes at the firehouse. One reminds you of another and you just roll with them.

Sunday mornings were the slowest time for us—all right, a little slower. It seemed that people were probably still passed out or hiding from the cops after a big Saturday night. I didn't care because I was usually a little hung over myself.

"GONG."

"Medic 16, respond, 1211 East Thirty-Second Street, for a possible DOA. Police en route," echoed the voice that broke a serene quiet. It wasn't unusual to get calls like this early in the morning. People that pass away in their sleep are found by their loved ones the next morning. I know this will sound sick but we had a few sayings referring to them. One was, "Start your day with a DOA" or "He must have woke up dead." I know what you're thinking and you're right. We arrived in front of the home located in the neighborhood near Lake Montibello and the famous Memorial Stadium. It was a modest area of well-kept, but old rowhomes. Doug and I casually walked to the front door and were greeted by a grieving man in his thirties. He told us that his father was dead and in the bedroom at the top of the stairs. A rather large woman, the deceased's wife, was sitting at the kitchen table crying into a dishtowel.

The steps creaked as Doug followed me up the stairs. An AM radio was blaring a Sunday gospel program in the first room we came to. The door was closed so we assumed it was the next room down the hall. The second door we came to had a hasp and padlock on it. We went back to the first door and slowly pushed it open. A small, frail looking, old man was lying in the bed. He looked very peaceful. I turned the radio down. The sheet and blanket were pulled up to his chin so only his head was visible, almost like the family had prepared him for our arrival. I reached down and grabbed the covers and whipped them back to expose the corpse. In a flash, he sat bolt upright and looked at me with his eyes popping out of his head. I jumped back and almost knocked Doug through the door.

"Jesus Christ!" I exclaimed.

"Why you botherin' me?" the now-lively corpse asked me, in a soft tone. Doug was laughing so hard I though he was going to collapse. I didn't find the humor in it because I was pissed.

"You're family thought you were dead for God's sake!" I blasted.

"I wunt det. Jus' sleepin'," he replied.

"Praise Jesus, thank you, Gawd!" exclaimed his wife, who was halfway up the stairs. For reasons beyond my comprehension, he refused to wake up for his family. Maybe he didn't feel like going to church today.

A Light at the End of the Tunnel

About five months had passed since the news of Matt's newfound employment. I had seen him at the pub a few times and was tired of hearing about fire school and his assignment after graduation from the academy.

I went to work one morning in February of 1985. Dan, from the off-going shift, told me that a guy from Medic 15 had been transferred to the new vacancy at Medic 9. Mine was the only transfer in for that spot when I filed it. That was my spot and I was on the phone to the duty officer in a flash. The next call would be to my union shop steward to file a grievance. The news I got from the lieutenant was wonderful!

It seems that a division chief from Anne Arundel County's Emergency Medical Services had gone to headquarters last week and requested a copy of my files. Was I in? That must have been the reason they denied my transfer because they knew I was gone.

On February 12, 1985, I received my letter of acceptance to the Anne Arundel County Fire Department. I called the EMS office and gave my notice that March 1st would be my last shift. No more Medic 16? Was it true? I was walking on a cloud and couldn't believe I had finally made it. Fire Recruit Class

Twenty-One wasn't starting until the last week of July but the county wanted me to report on March 7th. I didn't know or care why. The important part was—I was going home.

Chapter 11
Welcome, Rookie

The last two weeks in the city were long ones. It was hard to believe I was finally leaving and I'd never have to respond to the call, "Medic 16, Medic 16," again.

There wasn't a lot of hoopla amongst my friends, either. Doug and Jim were poking fun at me. I knew they were happy that I was moving on with my career but weren't happy that I was leaving them.

The firefighters usually got "pied" on their last shift, if they were transferring to a different station, or retiring. It's an age-old tradition in most departments. You get a, surprise, pie pan full of whipped cream mashed into your face when you least expect it. You look for it the whole shift but they always manage to get you by surprise. I got a couple of handshakes and hugs and that was it. I know that a couple of them were glad to see me go and I wouldn't miss them either.

I had called the county's office of personnel with some questions about my upcoming employment. They advised me that I was being hired as a lateral-entry paramedic, meaning that it was a transfer of certification as a CRT but my continued employment would be contingent on the successful completion of the fire academy class. I would report to the EMS office on March 7th. They would take me to the quartermaster's office where I'd be outfitted with everything I needed to do the job. This meant uniforms, a complete set of new turnout gear, dress shoes, work boots—the whole ten yards. I was excited.

I'd go through a two-week orientation to familiarize me with operating procedures within the department. Of course, being a former volunteer, I was already up to speed with response and radio procedures and having lived in the county for almost ten years, knew my way around pretty well.

My start date arrived and I was sitting in the parking lot of fire department headquarters an hour early. My hands were sweating and I had butterflies in my stomach. This was the first day of my new career. I was going to be wearing the uniform I'd dreamed of for years. I waited for some others to arrive and walked in with them. I knew a couple from the volunteer medic unit.

The biggest surprise was the arrival of my friend, Paul. He was a country boy from western Maryland who had worked with me in the city. He was on the shift that relieved me at Medic 16 but "burned out" after only six months. I hadn't seen him since his last shift there, almost a year earlier. We were cutting up about the great escape we had made from the city and some of the "prime" equipment we had while we were there. I wondered to myself if he would be able to handle the calls here, even though there were fewer of them. I guess time would tell but burnout is burnout. I never knew or heard of anyone that recovered from it.

Honestly, it doesn't take long to find out whether you're cut out for this profession or not. It can wear on you quickly, if you let it. Whenever someone would suddenly quit the service or do something crazy to get themselves off of a medic unit, I'd think about how lucky I was to have people like Louie and Cuz in my life. I had the power to overcome the little things that would eat away at my emotions or the big ones, called SEE's, by the experts (Significant Emotional Events)—at least I thought I did. If I ever had a problem dealing with them, I had people I could turn to.

After a few hours of filling out forms, photocopying ID's, and eye-drying informational talks, we headed for the quartermaster's office, down the hall. There were fourteen of us.

All This and a Bag of Chips

We were lined up in alphabetical order according to our last names and, as I stood there, thought of all the old movies I had seen where military draftees were doing the same thing. I laughed inside. This was great compared to the city where all they gave you were uniforms and a hard hat. It was my turn. The firefighter behind the counter verified my name.

"Praycheck," he said.

"It's Praschak," I replied.

"Whatever," he denounced. He asked for my shirt, pants, jacket, and shoe size. I wrote them on the form that would be used anytime I returned with garments that needed replacing (hopefully, because I wore them out and not because I "porked" out of them).

He returned with six long-sleeve and six short-sleeve work shirts, six work pants, a matching work jacket, a winter coat (called a Blauer jacket), a pair of combat boots with zippers up the sides, and a pair of work shoes that would double as my dress shoes. The Blauer was impressive with its removable liner and fuzzy collar. All the shirts and jackets had the county fire department and Maryland CRT patches sewn on them. Someone had asked about a Class A uniform or "dress blues." The reply was that the county had stopped issuing them a couple of years ago. I felt pretty proud and excited and even fumbled a little as I tried my shirts and jackets on for size. They fit me in more ways than one. The quartermaster then returned with three sets of AA and FD collar pins and, surprisingly, three chrome nameplates with my name on them—spelled correctly. I was impressed. Last, but not least, was the one item that I would take the most pride in. Hopefully I'd carry it with me for the rest of my career. It was my badge—number 435.

Next came the turnout gear. It was still in the factory plastic bags and boxes. A Cairns 880 helmet with face shield, short boots, turnout coat, turnout pants, a Nomex hood for under the helmet, firefighting gloves, leather work gloves, a yellow hard hat, and safety glasses were the order. I was in heaven. The final articles issued to us would have lasting effects on our memories and do, to this day. We were all issued t-shirts, gym shorts, long- and short-sleeve coveralls, and SPATS. Spats are white cotton, lace-up, ankle covers you see worn by most military academy recruits and some nostalgic or "throw-back" military uniforms. The instructions they gave with them were direct and simple. DO NOT WEAR YOUR SPATS, COVERALLS, OR GYM SHORTS UNTIL YOU REPORT TO THE ACADEMY FOR RECRUIT TRAINING. That was easy enough, but left me wondering what was ahead.

We hauled our booty to our vehicles and returned to the EMS office to get our station assignments. This was exciting, too. Where were they going to send me? Close to home, I hoped. The county is 485 square miles in area with more accessible shoreline than any county in the country, thanks to the Chesapeake Bay and five major tributaries. The city of Baltimore and Baltimore County border it to the north, Howard County to the west, and Calvert County to the south. The Chesapeake Bay borders the entire east side and the county encompasses the state capital of Annapolis, which has their own small department. I'll tell you more about the Annapolis Fire Department later.

The Envelope, Please

"Praycheck..." the lieutenant inquired.

"It's Praschak, sir," I repeated.

"Whatever. You're going to 31-B," he chirped.

"Thirty-one B—thank you, sir," I replied. Thirty-one—that figured. The station in Brooklyn was also known as the "Corner of 'What's Happenin' Now?'" It was the station closest to Baltimore city and wasn't much different, other than the location. When the city's Medics 9 and 5 were out at the same time, they would call on the county for assistance. This is known throughout the country as "Mutual Aid." Paramedic 31 spent more time in the city than any other north county unit and would actually transport patients to city hospitals that were closer than the main hospital in North County. I just can't get out of hell, can I? I guess, realizing I was fresh from the "jungle," the county wanted to ease me back into society and dealing with "human beings." Oh well, it was still a step forward and getting hired by the county gave me a $6,000-a-year raise over what I had been making in the city.

Brooklyn earned its nickname because it seemed that there was always something going on outside the firehouse, and someone working there was always asking "What's happening now?" as they ran to the window to investigate. It was, technically, a volunteer station and one of the originals in the county, dating back to the early 1930s. There were no active members these days other than an administrative board that maintained the building and paid the utility bills. There was an engine, truck, paramedic unit, and reserve ambulance housed there. It was one of the few stations where everyone there was a career firefighter.

The county had three stations that were owned and staffed by the county and located in areas that the dwindling volunteer staff couldn't cover or where call volumes had increased due to population and business increases.

I was going to 31 on "B" shift and was going to be working with a paramedic they called Rob. He was a Viet Nam combat veteran and in the fire department for seven years, after transferring from public works. You could do that here. My first couple of shifts were stressful. I had my little habits that had to be broken, like carrying my personal aid bag with me. After two calls, Rob had had enough.

"Lose the bag, Rookie!" he barked as we arrived at a call. "You're in the county now, they supply the shit. Lose it," he enforced. But, I loved my bag and I'm not a rookie. I knew what Linus felt like when Snoopy snatched his blanket, now, and how many times do I have to be a rookie in my life?

I was nervous and knew the time had come, once again, for me to prove myself. It seemed like I was doing that a lot in this profession. About a month had passed and I was getting to know Rob better. I felt like he was tolerating me better, too. I had the feeling, initially, that he wasn't happy about getting one of the rookies.

Waaaahhhhh…

The Claxon horn in the station blared. Unlike the city with its traditional gong and watch desk, the county stations had no watch desk and an electronic alert system. Think of the television show *EMERGENCY*.

"Medical Box 31-8, Engine and Paramedic 31 respond to the Value City, 6128 Ritchie Highway, for a cardiac arrest—CPR in progress," came the call. This was the first cardiac arrest that Rob and I would handle together. Station 31 was located on Ritchie Highway so it was a straight shot, about four miles down the road. As we arrived, an employee of the store directed us in. We loaded our gear on the stretcher and rolled in, through the racks of clothes, to the men's department.

There, in between racks, was one of our off-duty paramedics, working CPR alone. He looked tired. I immediately got the elder valve set up and handed it to one of the firefighters from the engine. The other firefighter took over chest compressions. It was nice having them right there to assist, as opposed to having to call and wait for them to get there. Rob and I could do our thing now, without a delay.

I cut the elderly man's shirt off of him and applied the electrode pads for the EKG to his chest. He had very little chest hair so it was easy to get them to stick. Sometimes you had to be a freakin' barber first, shaving the spots where the electrodes are placed, so they'd stick. Women were never a problem (well, most women).

Rob was setting up for the IV and I quickly snapped the esophageal obturator airway (EOA) together, lubed the end, and inserted it in the patient's mouth. The tube has a mask on one end and the inflatable balloon or cuff on the other end. The firefighter now had a good airway to work with and only needed to assure a good seal with the mask on the patient's face. I glanced at the EKG screen and noticed that the patient was in coarse ventricular fibrillation. We needed to shock him right away.

Coarse v-fib is the rhythm that most heart attack victims go into initially and a lot of times you get good results if you can shock them early enough to restore a reasonably normal rhythm. This fact was realized by the medical field and, nowadays, first responders (including police officers) carry AED's or automatic external defibrillators. They're found in places of business everywhere and most commonly found in restaurants and on commercial aircraft.

You can probably thank Ray, the off-duty medic, for his rapid response and CPR in keeping the patient's condition from deteriorating before we got there. CPR is a lifesaver and I never understood why it wasn't a required course for every student, from grade school on. I removed the paddles from the EKG monitor and applied some conductive gel to them. Not only did the gel increase electrical conductivity but reduced the burn on the patient's chest. I hit the "charge" button for 200 joules (the first measurement of voltage we'd deliver).

Wheeeeeeeeeee.......BEEP. The paddles were charged. I held them tight against the man's chest, in position.

"CLEAR," I ordered. The firefighters stopped CPR and backed off. If you've ever been, or seen someone, in contact with a body that's being shocked, you know to do this. Each paddle had a trigger and they had to be depressed at the same time. "ZAP!" The man's body was jolted and the screen on the EKG went blank, which was normal. It would restore itself in seconds and the waiting seemed like minutes. The line returned to the screen but there were no changes. The firefighters resumed CPR and we had to shock him again, this time at 300 joules. I recharged the unit.

"CLEAR," I repeated. ZAP! There were still no changes. One more shock at 360 joules, then Rob would stick him (start the IV). After three unsuccessful shocks, the IV would be started and the first round of drugs would be administered. We'd give him a milligram of Epinephrine (adrenaline) and a dose of Lidocaine, calculated by his weight—probably seventy-five milligrams. CPR is then continued for a couple minutes to circulate the medications. I charged the unit for the third time. "CLEAR," I again ordered. ZAP.

"WE GOT SOMETHIN', ROB. See if you've got a pulse with this," I said enthusiastically, as the screen returned. It was a rhythm—slow, but a rhythm nonetheless. Rob slid two fingers onto the man's neck and checked for a carotid pulse. The firefighters were positioned to resume CPR if necessary.

"It's weak but it's there," Rob announced. Awesome! The patient wasn't breathing on his own but at least we had his heart beating again. It was a good start and too many times it's been three shocks, all the drugs, and nothing. This felt pretty good. Rob got the IV in and pushed the first round of drugs. The Epi would increase the patient's blood pressure, heart rate, and the force of the heart's contractions. The Lidocaine would help keep the lethal rhythm from recurring. The Epi worked right away. The patient's heart rate increased to near normal. All the time, we checked for any kind of movement in his extremities or eye movement. If you're not ready, and an unconscious patient wakes up, the first thing he wants to do is rip the tube out of his mouth, like my "druggies" in the city.

Sure enough, ten minutes after shocking this man back "from the dead," his fingers began to move—then his hands—then his arms.

"HOLD HIM DOWN!" I exclaimed, as each firefighter got a wrist. One of the best feelings I've had in this business, so far, was seeing this man open his eyes. It was better than hearing the first cries of a newborn. I realized that I had just cheated the Grim Reaper and given this person's family their loved one back. There are a few things to understand, though. Most people that are revived after cardiac arrest usually don't live long afterwards or have a poor prognosis. The quality of their life is changed and a lot end up in nursing homes. I guess the bottom line is, they could have been planning his funeral and now can pray for him to recover. Sometimes praying is all that we have left, but it's something.

We tied the man's wrists to the backboard and I bent over to talk to him. I got close to his ear and in a soft, but authoritative voice, assured him that he was going to be all right. I explained to him what had just happened and told him I was removing the tube, and it would be easier to tolerate if he relaxed as much as possible. I think he understood me because the words seemed to keep him calm. A tear ran from his eye, down his cheek. I'm not sure if it was a tear of sadness from what had occurred or the happiness of just being alive. It didn't really matter. I wiped it away for him.

Two weeks later a basket of fruit arrived at the station. It was addressed to "All that helped save my husband's life." We recognized the last name. Along with the fruit was a card that explained that her husband had made a miraculous recovery and was now resting at home, thanks to us.

This was what my job was all about—saving lives. I wish it happened more often because the feeling I had after this call was euphoric, beyond your imagination. As I sat at the desk in the station's paramedic office, processing the previous day's reports, Rob walked in with the card in his hand.

"Not bad for a fuckin' rookie," he said, as he smiled, tossed the card on the desk, and walked away. I think I just made the grade again.

Keep Your Cool

There were times in the past, when I'd go to a call and have confrontations with patients, for one reason or another. They were not heated arguments and a lot had to do with convincing a person that they needed medical attention when they thought otherwise. More times than not, they were with family members who thought they could call the shots. The law that governs Emergency Services personnel is well defined and we're constantly reminded that by our superiors. This was especially true if a patient or family member would file a complaint because they thought we had not acted prudently or overstepped our boundaries.

I was well-versed in the legal aspect of my job, and my duties and limitations. I was always sympathetic to the needs of my patients and their families. If I was confronted, I stood my ground in a manner that was always professional. I knew what I was talking about. Having control of your emotions was probably one of the most important skills you could possess in this business but keep in mind—we're human, too. I had a reminder before leaving Brooklyn.

Waaaaaaaaaahhhh….

"Rescue Box 31-6, Engine 31, Truck 31, Paramedic 31, Ambulance 34, EMS 3, Battalion Chief 1 respond for an auto accident with entrapment, Baltimore-Annapolis Boulevard at the overpass to I-695, cross street Hammonds Lane," was the call.

Calls like these really get your adrenaline going. Every second counts on a lot of calls, especially rescues of any type. Rob and I were the first ones out the door which meant we'd be the first ones to arrive unless 34, or either the EMS duty officer or chief responding, happened to be on the road and closer. As we approached the scene we could see that it was a nasty crash.

We left room for the truck to get close since they had the rescue tools on board. A jacked-up four-wheel-drive pickup had apparently crossed the centerline and struck a Pacer head-on, on the bridge. The lift kit on the pickup allowed its front bumper to clear the hood of the Pacer. The female driver of the Pacer was pinned, badly.

I had my coat and helmet on in no time, grabbed the aid bag and oxygen, and crawled into the Pacer through the back window, which had popped open on impact. The victim was still breathing, but barely. She had a massive facial injury and blood was entering her airway with every breath. Rob had seen this and was quick to get a suction unit to me through the passenger side window. I placed gauze pads on her face, around her mouth and nose, to slow the blood flow and try to get a seal on the mask of the pressure ventilator. Her face was disfigured so badly I had to try to build some kind of foundation to get some air in her. I had a bad feeling. *Where's the Hurst tool?* I thought to myself. Normally I'd hear the tool running by now. The "Jaws of Life" had distinct sound. It was the sound of death in some cases—the sound of life in others. It was never a good sound.

"ROB, WHERE'S THE FUCKIN' TOOL?" I shouted from within.

"They're trying to get it started. Sorry, bud. Thirty-Two's on the way with a second one. Hang in there," he encouraged. I wasn't the one that needed to "hang in there," the victim was. I had a habit of talking to patients, even the unconscious ones. Encouragement helps on every call and no one can say whether they can hear you or not.

"Hang in there, baby. We're doing the best we can for ya'." I spoke softly into her ear. I really felt helpless as Rob started an IV in the patient's arm, through the driver's side window. I kept breathing for her and occasionally checking her carotid pulse (in her neck). I could only imagine what other injuries were beneath the wreckage once she was free.

Truck 32 finally arrived and just as the lieutenant from the truck stuck his head through the window, I lost the seal on the victim's face and blood sprayed everywhere. It splashed my face and all over his white uniform shirt. He should have had his turnout coat buttoned, anyway, and it didn't bother me. I kept working—sweating, cramping in my thighs and hands, trying to keep this lady alive. Rob reached in and swabbed the blood off my face.

I heard the pump running for the rescue tool—thank God. It would be a good fifteen minutes to half an hour to get her free, once the tool got in service. It seemed like I had been in there for an hour. Rob threw a rescue blanket in and covered us up to prevent us from getting hit with flying glass or shrapnel from the working tool.

Finally, I felt the pressure relief on the patient. The door was gone and the dash pried away from her. I knew we were getting close and Rob and the guys outside had a backboard under her ass, as I felt her move.

"We got her, Mark." Rob said. I just lay there after she was removed—spent. Two firefighters from the engine helped me out the back. I went right to Rob's side and a med-evac helicopter was waiting for her. I never even heard them arrive. Rob and I continued supporting the victim's airway as a medic from Paramedic 18 secured her to the board. I never knew they were there, either. I checked for a pulse on the victim, one last time, before we headed for the chopper.

"FUCK, ROB, SHE'S IN ARREST," I shouted, as I started chest compressions with one hand. She had gone into cardiac arrest. I was surprised she had lasted this long but hoped she had made it a little longer. We pushed drugs through the IV and did CPR along the way to the waiting med-evac. I staggered up the grade as the helicopter flew off. As I approached the wreckage that I got so personal with, I noticed 34 with a teenage girl on their stretcher, heading toward their unit.

"Where'd she come from?" I inquired.

"She was a passenger in the car, that was her mom. We were just waiting for you to finish," stated the volly EMT.

"SHE WAS IN THAT CAR?" I shouted. The volly nodded as he continued on. It was a miracle because she had a couple of large scratches on her leg and arm, but that was it.

Just then, I heard a guy sitting on the guardrail say, "HEY, WHEN IS SOMEONE GONNA TAKE CARE OF ME?" His nose was swollen and looked like it was broken. I was told by one of the rescue workers that he was the driver of the pickup, he was drunk, and they had found some weed in his truck. It was then that I lost my cool, for the first time ever.

I charged over to him, grabbed his shirt with both hands, and picked him up off the guardrail. I almost had his feet off the ground.

"YOU MOTHERFUCKER, YOU JUST KILLED A WOMAN AND HER DAUGHTER SAT NEXT TO HER AND WATCHED. YOU WANT HELP? I'LL GIVE YOU SOME HELP," I raged. The battalion chief and a firefighter had to pry my hands from the guy. I tried head-butting him just as they got us apart, but was too late. A cop had me by my belt and the three quickly dragged me away.

"I'LL KICK YOUR ASS, YOU SORRY MOTHERFUCKER," I shouted, as they dragged me away from him. I would have, too, had they not been there.

"MARK, MARK" Chief James shouted, as he grabbed me in a manner that I had just displayed. He was a big man and knew me from my volly days, and I think he used to like me.

"Gather your shit up and go. I know how you're feeling. Just go to 26 and clean up there. We'll talk later," he said sternly. I relaxed and tried to comprehend what had just happened in the last two minutes. I'd never been here before. I couldn't believe I lost control like that. *NOT ME—THE WORLD'S BEST MEDIC.* I had problems now. Was he going to fire me or suspend me? I was a probationary firefighter. Was this the end of the line? I was silent until we got to 26. Rob was, too. I think he was pissed at me but I didn't care and I thought about Cuz, my mentor. How would he have handled the situation? I felt like I had let down everyone that helped me get here. I wanted to cry.

Crisis Intervention

I had learned about "crisis intervention" a long time ago. After all, it's what we did on almost every call in one aspect or another. I didn't think that we, as "service" workers, would ever need it. Hell, it was for other people.

We arrived at Station 26 and Rob went inside. I stayed outside and tried to start cleaning equipment. I could only imagine what he said about me in there, but I still didn't care. It was hard to focus on a task because I had this call on my mind. I found myself doing five things at once. I couldn't complete one task without becoming distracted and starting another. The funny thing was, I didn't realize what was happening at the time. I heard the door to the station open.

"Hey, what's up?" a voice came. It was Alan, one of the senior paramedics in the department. He was also an instructor I had met at a lecture he did (Crisis Intervention) while I was in CRT school.

"Not much," I said, shortly.

"Heard you had a rough one," he said.

"Yeah, it was ugly," I returned. I really wasn't up for small talk.

"Wanna talk about it?" he asked.

"Not much to talk about, I fucked up. Probably gonna lose my job," I said.

"Nah, you're not the first one that's had a problem and won't be the last either," he reinforced. I couldn't help myself and a tear ran down my cheek. I loved my job and I didn't want it to end, especially like this.

"Doc said you did a helluva job in that car up there," he claimed. I looked at him with a bewildered look.

"Yeah? I guess I blew it, though," I said with a sniffle.

"Hey, I've been there. We all have. Sometimes people make you want to do shit like that. You just have to bite your tongue and walk away. I know it's tough sometimes but I had to learn just like you did," he said. This guy was good. I felt better already and I needed this. I didn't feel like I was alone anymore. The "cold shoulder" from Rob, on the way here, had isolated me. I felt like I was coming back from a "bad" place.

"I've never done anything like that, EVER, and believe me the city had some that needed to be jacked up," I spoke.

"Like I said, you're gonna have one's that push you to your limit. Deal with it! I know you can do it because I've heard a lot about your work. We need good medics like you, the question is, how good do you want to be?" he questioned.

"Don't ask yourself how good you are, just BE good," he added. Was he bullshitting me or did he really hear about my work? Regardless, it was making me feel better. What about the chief?

"That's good advice, Al, but maybe, too late," I said.

"(Chief) James called me and said he was sending you here. He told me that if I thought you had a real problem, we'd take it from there. I don't think you have a problem. I think you just learned a lesson that we all learn when we get started in this business. I think you'll be fine. Just learn from it and move on, bro." he said. I shook his hand.

"Thanks, Alan, I needed this," I said, graciously.

"I know you did and you'll be OK," he finished. He walked back toward the station and I went back to work, relieved.

The Funniest Thing I Ever Saw

We had a lieutenant, named Lenny, that used to love working overtime at 31. He was assigned to Communications when he got promoted but really wanted to work in the field, more than anything. He was a nut and I loved working and playing ball with him. He was one of the funniest people I ever met.

There was a restaurant on the adjacent corner across from the firehouse. We called it "The Rant" because the "Restau" letters in the neon sign were always flashing or out completely—leaving just the "rant" lit. There was a Metro bus stop on the corner there, along with a phone booth, and a couple of newspaper vending boxes. It was a busy bus stop and seemed to have people waiting at all hours of the day and night. One day, Lenny approached me in the office and said, "Come here, watch this."

All the other guys on the shift had gathered in the lounge that overlooked the front, and "Rant-side" of the building. There were four people waiting at the bus stop. Lenny picked up the phone on the end table and dialed.

"What are we doing?" I asked, innocently.

"Just watch," the group insisted. Lenny was calling the pay phone in the phone booth at the bus stop. After a minute or two of ringing, one of the men at the stop answered it.

"Yes, this is the MTA [Maryland Transportation Authority] calling. I want to let you know that Bus 14 is running late by about fifteen minutes. If you want to go into the restaurant and have a refreshment, get a receipt and the driver will reimburse you when the bus arrives," Lenny said in a professional tone. We were pissing our pants, trying not to let the guy on the other end hear us laughing. When Lenny hung up, we burst out in laughter. Now, to see if we had any takers. We could see the guy talking to the other riders. All at once, the three men headed for the Rant, leaving the only woman behind. She was the smart one, I guessed. Sure enough, two minutes later, Bus 14 rolled up. The door opened and the woman climbed aboard. The three men ran out of the Rant, but too late. The doors on the bus closed and it pulled away. I thought I was going to die. I never laughed so hard in my life.

A couple of weeks later, Lenny joined us for another shift. We talked about the last shift, when we made the riders miss the bus, and had another laugh. He had another one up his sleeve. After housework was done, we gathered in the lounge again. It was a Sunday morning and there was one man at the bus stop. Lenny picked up the phone and called him but it rang and rang. The guy wouldn't pick it up and we were bumming. Lenny let it ring and finally, the guy bit.

"YEAH, TOMMY, IT'S ME. THE MONEY IS UNDER THE PAPERS, JUST LIKE WE PLANNED," Lenny said, excitedly. The guy questioned him.

"JUST GET THE FUCKIN' MONEY AND MEET ME, LIKE WE PLANNED. IT'S UNDER THE PAPERS!" Lenny insisted, just before he abruptly hung the phone up. I was having chest pains—I was laughing so hard. Tears were rolling down my face and my sides were aching. The guy came out of the phone booth and lit a cigarette. He was looking around and looked really nervous. He dug in his pocket, apparently looking for four quarters for the Sunday paper. Suddenly he trots towards the Rant. I guess he needed change.

After a minute, he trots out of the Rant, and directly to the first paper box. He put his money in the box, opened the door, and started pulling the papers out. He was stacking them, neatly, on the ground next to the box. We were NO GOOD. I'm surprised he couldn't hear the eight of us laughing. I never realized how many BIG Sunday papers that were in one of those boxes.

After removing the papers and not finding the treasure, he loaded them back into the box, closed the door, and lit another cigarette. Was he going to try the other box? Did he have enough change for that one? Should he chance it? What do you think? He puffed away on his cigarette. Sure enough, he headed back to the Rant for another round of quarters. While he was inside, Bus 14 steamed by and up the hill. I didn't think I could laugh any harder, but I did. The guy came out and stopped, dead in his tracks, as he watched the bus disappear up Ritchie Highway. We couldn't read his lips but could tell he was pissed. We couldn't have timed it more perfectly. This was like watching a silent comedy on TV, but it was really happening. Oh well, time to collect the booty.

He walked over to the second paper box and put his money in. He opened the door and started pulling the papers out. He wasn't very tidy this time and just threw them on the ground as fast as he could pull them out. After the last paper hit the ground, he stuck his head inside the box only to find that, not only was there no treasure, but he missed his bus, and it cost him two dollars. He slammed the door of the paper box so hard, it shook the light post that it was chained to. He lit another cigarette as he stomped away in the direction of the bus, leaving twenty Sunday papers scattered in front of the Rant. That was the first and only time I laughed so hard, I needed oxygen afterwards.

Rob and I worked together at 31 for the next two months until I got moved to the "Heights," where a vacancy needed to be filled. Fire School starts in three weeks.

Chapter 12
Boot Camp

The Heights was a, primarily, volunteer station. They had one of the larger volunteer memberships and was located near some pretty exclusive neighborhoods and businesses, so donations were plentiful. They could afford a lot of nice equipment that they bought, with the county's blessing of course. There was a career engineman, a day-work firefighter and two career paramedics on each shift, similar to the volunteer station I had started at, here in the county—less the paid medic unit.

I was assigned to Station 12, "B" shift and was working on Paramedic 12 with two guys named Ron and Sherman. Ron was a twenty-year-plus veteran whose reputation preceded him (I was warned ahead of time). He was a "bad boy" and seemed to be proud of those incidents that had earned him his badge, judging from the way he bragged about being brought up on departmental charges. I wasn't impressed.

He was a short-timer (had less than ten years till retirement) and was, basically, just here for the money. He lacked any motivation to promote, even to the rank of EMT-P (let alone officer). He despised anyone with "bugles." Officers in the fire department wore collar pins that brandished old fire department horns that those in charge used to shout orders on the fireground through—similar to those used by cheerleading squads. That was in the days before radio systems. More commonly called bugles, a lieutenant had pins with one bugle, a captain two, a battalion chief three, a deputy chief four, and the chief of the department, five. That being said, Ron hated them all. His analysis of his job description was, "drive truck, get check." Sherman, on the other hand, seemed pretty laid back—aloof at times. I was more comfortable working with him. He was easier to work with and I didn't worry about being tagged in part of some conspiracy with him, like I felt when I worked with Ron. Either way, they both knew their protocols and had good skills and hopefully could teach me things other than how to avoid being brought down by "the system."

Waaaaaaah…

"Medical Box 20-4, Engine 20, Paramedic 12 respond for a person with trouble breathing at number 2124 Chelsea Beach Road, cross street of Woods Road," came the call. I had been working at 12 for about three weeks and had mostly routine calls and nothing to write a book about. Engine 20 arrived first and a firefighter met us on the street as we arrived.

"We got us a big one, fellas," he advised.

"Big one? How big?" Sherman inquired as we dragged our equipment from their places.

"Oh, five maybe six," he said calmly.

"HUNDRED?" I gasped.

"Not ounces, Rookie," he returned. Everyone knew who the rookies were, it seemed.

Holy shit, he wasn't kidding. This was the biggest person I had ever seen. My head was spinning and this guy was in bad shape. It was warm, humid spring weather, which always brought out the asthmatics and "breathers" (people with COPD or chronic obstructive pulmonary disease).

The crew from the engine had put nasal oxygen on the patient, thinking they would cause him greater distress if they gave him a higher concentration, which is true for some patients that have a low oxygen level in their blood normally. This guy's skin was ashen—he was sweating profusely, and barely moving air. It was pretty obvious that he had been getting worse, as opposed to getting better, over the last several hours. I switched him to a high-concentration mask.

Most people with chronic medical problems hate going to the doctor's office, hate the hospital, and even hate calling 911, because they do it so often. Most just wait, thinking they might get better on their own, which is almost never the case. When they get worse we have a handful and in this case we had a truckload. It took all five of us to get this guy from the couch to the stretcher when we made a painful discovery. We couldn't get him through the doorway, or ANY doorway in the entire house, for that matter. He was too wide. Hell, we couldn't see the stretcher with him on it. We needed more help, so let's start a squad. The call came out.

"Medical Box 20-4, Squad 12 respond to assist Engine 20 and Paramedic 12 with trouble breathing, number 2124 Chelsea Beach Road, cross street,

Woods Road. Respond Priority 1." Sherman and I had done all the advanced life support for the patient by the time the squad arrived. It was apparent that we couldn't fit enough people in the room to physically lift him up so the plan was to get him on a salvage cover (tarp) and drag him outside, then get him back on the stretcher, somehow. Now, to make the opening bigger. The crew on the squad started by removing the kitchen door, which was the closest. We measured it but no dice—it was still not wide enough. Now, without tearing up too much we'd remove the door frame but keep in mind, the man's going downhill, fast. Five minutes later with the door frame removed eight of us wedged the whale-like body through the opening. The next back-breaking task would be to get him on the stretcher and lifted into the medic unit. Remember, also, we couldn't even see the stretcher with him on it, let alone find a lifting point—stop, I have an idea.

"Fuck the stretcher, we use the kitchen door as a ramp and drag the whole works into the back of the unit. The squad can take our stretcher, meet us at the hospital, and help us unload him," I ordered. That was BRILLIANT and it worked (although they do need a new kitchen door). Not bad for a rookie, huh? The patient, who's suffered from his chronic disease for fifteen years, died two weeks later. I'm having mixed emotions, now. I feel somewhat relieved that the poor man isn't suffering anymore, but ask myself if my actions didn't prolong his suffering. I may need the help of my mentors on this one.

FALL IN!

July 27, 1985, was a day that will go down in infamy, as my first day in hell.

"CLASS 21, FALL IN, FOUR ROWS, ARM'S LENGTH APART. MOVE, YOU ROOKIES," shouted an instructor to thirty-five poor souls in t-shirts, gym shorts, and running shoes.

TEN-SHUN. ROLL CALL," he orders. A few minutes pass before he calls my name.

"PRAYCHECK"

"IT'S PRASCHAK, SIR," I demanded.

"WHATEVER," he says. What's up with these people?

"COUNT OFF IN FOURS," he ordered. We were broken down into four "squads." Each squad had a recruit that was a military veteran as their "squad leader." The age range of our class was from twenty to forty-five (yes, there was a forty-five-year-old man about to enter hell, so this ought to be good). I would be thirty in three months.

I knew that the majority of the class that had been taking basic EMT for three weeks had been running during the physical training (PT) portion of the class first thing every morning. Fourteen lateral-entry paramedics had just joined the festivities. I had been running about a mile every day to get conditioned. The class was already up to two miles a day and I thought I was going to die. Satan wrote the physical training exercises himself. Pushups, situps, jumping jacks, leg lifts (til' your abdomen burned), and our all-time favorite, arm twirls (until they felt like they were going to fall off) were on the menu. If you couldn't do them or did them poorly, you had an instructor barking in your face till you did. Four instructors encircled our group for quality control. I do not like this and it's only the first day.

"NOW LET'S GO FOR A RUN, YOU MAGGOTS," one instructor ordered. These instructors knew how to abuse because they put the longest legs in the front of the group. This meant that those of us that were more vertically challenged (I'm five feet, ten inches, but have short legs) were running our asses off. I dropped back after the first mile, as did my paramedic counterparts. How can someone run backwards and holler in your face at the same time? It's possible because I experienced it.

After running to what seemed like Baltimore and back, we were ordered to the showers. The locker rooms and shower facility were located in the headquarters building and not at the actual training facility. We had to fall-in, in formation, in fifteen minutes with coveralls, spats, and hardhats. There were three, 360-degree showers with stainless catch basins. We gathered around them like broken inmates in some foreign prison. Some had to stand, naked, waiting their turn. I wanted to stand there for an hour but God forbid if I was late for formation. I only imagined.

I didn't feel bad after I was showered and dressed, standing at ease, waiting for the next round of abuse. I felt silly wearing the spats but I didn't dare mention that. Now we got to march, in formation, a quarter-mile down the hill behind the headquarters building, to the training academy. We'd be in the classroom in the morning and doing practical work after lunch. We'd bag our lunch, or go hungry, because there's no leaving hell till the end of the day. I survived Day 1 as my weary ass limped to my car. I got home at five, was in bed by five-thirty, and asleep by five-thirty-five. Just think, only fifteen weeks and four days to go.

Suddenly, Things Change

I would miss the next week of class. I got home from class one evening, when my phone rang. It was my brother, in Cincinnati. He informed me that my mom had suffered a massive heart attack while her and my dad vacationed in Las Vegas. She was alive, but in intensive care, and they had implanted a temporary pacemaker. I knew it was serious and SHE BETTER NOT DIE.

I would fly to Cincinnati and meet my brother, then we'd both fly to Vegas from there. My uncle, who worked for American Airlines in Newark, New Jersey, for twenty-five years, booked our tickets. I was crying as I packed my bag but managed to gather myself long enough to make the call to Communications, instructing the supervisor to pass the word that I was going to miss class for an undetermined amount of time. At this point in time, I could care less about my job. I was always "Mama's Boy"—her first and oldest.

I was informed by the doctor that attended to Mom, that she had suffered an anterior wall, myocardial infarction—the deadliest kind. She was playing the slots at Caesar's Palace at 9:30 in the morning (I get my gambling bone from her) when she started feeling bad. Fortunately, Caesar's has a doctor's office in the hotel. She went to the room, woke my dad, and they went right to the office.

When I found out that this doctor at Caesar's didn't immediately call 911 and told them to take a cab to the hospital, I was ready to hunt him down and kick his ass. Fortunately she made it there and was given immediate attention. I was at the hospital every day for the next six days. What a helluva way to see Vegas for the first time. When the doctors felt Mom had gotten the strength enough to endure the flight, they sent her home. They instructed her to go directly to a cardiologist the day she arrived back home. She didn't get home until late but went to a cardiologist at the local hospital the next day. After a barrage of tests they admitted her.

The next day she had successful quadruple bypass surgery. I called Dad after class every night. Fortunately, working for the county for four months prior to the academy had allowed me to accrue enough sick leave to keep me from getting fired.

NFPA 1001

When I returned to class, we were told, within the next few days, that we were the first class in the history of the Anne Arundel County Fire Department being trained to meet the National Fire Protection Association's strict, 1001 Standards for Firefighting. This meant that we would be tested on a set of national standards and not the department's guidelines that had been followed since its inception in 1965.

We would have time limits on evolutions and distance running. We had required classes and tasks to meet that no other fire academy class had to, thus far. We also had something else that no other class had, either—an abundance of female recruits. There were three females in the department at the time. Times were changing and the law stated that we needed more. At the time, I had no problem with this. I thought, if they can survive this abuse and make the grade, that they deserve the job. Of the thirty-five recruits, nine were female. Let the games begin.

Our girls were taking a pounding by week two. One had twisted an ankle while running and another had a knee injury during an evolution. We're down to seven after only two weeks. No boys were out but some racial tensions were flaring. We had five or six black male recruits, and some of the white guys had issues with that. I wasn't worried because I got along with everyone regardless of his or her race, which has always been my nature. I only had a problem with my squad leader, but not because he was black. He was dumber than a "box of rocks" and our squad was running a lot of extra laps around the compound because of dumb shit he would do. If one in your squad screwed up, the whole squad paid for it.

From the first day of training, my friend and fellow lateral entry, Jimmy and I, were assigned to the flag detail. We formally marched the American and county flags to the pole at the entrance to the academy every morning and retrieved them at the end of the day, with the rest of the class standing in formation, at attention. One day, an instructor noticed that the flags weren't spaced to his liking. What? He interrupted the entire operation from whatever they were doing and made the whole class line up in formation.

"FLAG DETAIL, FALL OUT AND FIX MY FLAGS, DAMMIT," he ordered. Jimmy and I had to lower the flags to re-space them another two inches apart. Then, we all had to run a lap around the compound, some in full turnout gear. HEY, THEY WERE SPACED THE SAME AS ANY OTHER DAY, GIVE US A BREAK. That same instructor, CJ (a hard-assed tricky and former Marine DI) was assigned by the staff as the "enforcer." If you took one step into a building or garage with your cover (hardhat) on, POW, he got you. We tagged him as "The Agitator."

"PRAYCHECK, YOU OWE ME," he blasted. That meant I'd have to stay after dismissal and give him twenty pushups.

"It's Praschak, sir," I returned.

"WHATEVER, YOU OWE ME DOUBLE, NOW," he shouted. I didn't care because I was going to correct them until they got it right. Every day at roll call, it was the same routine. It was comical to everyone but me. Everyone else would acknowledge by saying "Here, sir," but not me.

"PRAYCHECK."

"IT'S PRASCHAK, SIR."

"WHATEVER." This went on every day, for sixteen weeks.

One day, about six weeks into the class, the racial tensions came to a head. It really boiled down to two guys, one black (my squad leader) and one white. They just didn't like each other. They had words in the locker room just before formation and were nose to nose. That's when a really cool thing happened. We became united and all intervened—blacks and whites. We knew we would all pay because the instructors had warned us about fighting and stressed how important "teamwork" and "family" were. Termination would be the result of fighting so we separated them and read them the "riot act." I was especially vocal, being one of the older guys in the class.

I felt like I had already gained some respect from the instructors because of my age and experience. They would give me tasks to lighten their load, for example in rope class while tying knots. I love rope work and had done truck work in almost every station I'd worked at. They all knew this and had me working with those in my squad that needed help. I was "volunteered" to tie a rescue knot (blindfolded) for the audience at the upcoming Fire Exposition that was held for the public each year during Fire Prevention Week. I nailed it like Houdini.

Every Friday evening, after our week of abuse, the majority of us would end up across the street at the local watering hole. It had become ritual and the bartender would have ten Buds and ten or fifteen Coors Light bottles opened and waiting for us at 5:15, like clockwork. One Friday, with four weeks to go until graduation, none other than CJ joined us. The place got so quiet, you'd have thought someone died. We all stood there looking at him as he stopped in his tracks with a blank look on his face. It was like twenty gunfighters looking at one, in a showdown. Some of the guys looked pissed, like he had invaded our sacred ground. Some just looked down, as if they had gotten caught doing something wrong. I just looked at him with this amazed look on my face. That guy had some pretty big stones to walk into that bar. He looked at me and got this shit-eating grin on his face as if to say "What, can't a man have a beer?"

I finally broke the silence. "GET THAT MAN A FUCKING BEER, ON ME," I ordered. He grinned from ear to ear and a cheer went out from the crowd. We all walked over to him and, one at a time, shook his hand. Did we have a friend or a spy? I guess we'd find out on Monday but in the meantime, there was beer to drink. We normally headed home before eleven but no one left that night. We shot pool and tossed darts all night and all closed the place at two—CJ included.

Monday morning roll call always came too soon and it was business as usual. CJ was back to being the agitating, pain-in-the-ass he normally was. That was the first and only time we'd see him at the bar, too.

Four to Go

With just four weeks left until graduation, the pressure to perform was building. Some were worried and the females were failing—all of them. None of them were completing the evolutions in time. We knew the staff was concerned and knew that the brass at the "Brick Shit House" (headquarters) were, too, because they spent a lot of time in the chief of training's office— sometimes for hours a day. It wasn't gonna be pretty if the women's times didn't improve. I was just doing my thing and my times improved with every practice evolution. One day we had to perform an evolution called the "Metro Bottle Change." The staff would charge the "dollhouse" with smoke until it was chugging out of the eaves like an old locomotive.

The "dollhouse" was the place where we trained for live fires and rescues. It was a two-story, Cape Cod, made of cinder blocks, concrete floors, and a steel roof. IT WAS HOT, especially when we did the basement fire evolution. There was also the "tower." It was a five-story building that had a fire escape on one side and a flat roof. We would do things like roof rescues and general truck and ladder work there. The staff would always make us deploy the "air bag" before we had any evolutions involving the tower. It was a twenty-by-twenty-foot bag about eight feet high, filled with air. We actually practiced jumping into it from the fourth floor one day. That was some of the only fun I can recall.

During the "Metro Bottle Change" evolution, we had to get in full turnout gear including SCBA. We would carry a spare SCBA air bottle with us, into the attic. Smoke and heat rise so you can imagine what the attic was like when smoke was pouring out the front door, on the first floor.

Once in the attic, we had to breathe air out of our original air bottle until the low air alarm bell started ringing. We would then remove our harness with the original air bottle in it, shut the old bottle down, remove it, install the new bottle, and put the harness back on. Think about this. When the low air alarm bell starts ringing, you have about five minutes of breathing air left. The harder you're breathing the less time you have. When you remove your harness and original bottle, you have to hold your breath while switching over to the new bottle— all in a hot, dark, and smoke-filled attic. You couldn't see your hand in front of your face if you tried and I know because I tried. My squad practiced outside the dollhouse, closing our eyes to simulate the conditions. I had it down but was a little scared.

Suddenly, the side door burst open and one of the instructors was dragging someone out. It was a black guy named Daniels. He must have freaked out and was coughing and throwing up. Another instructor arrived with an oxygen bottle and started pumping Daniels some fresh stuff. He took about five deep breaths, and yacked right on the instructor's boots. We were no good and all of us were laughing our asses off, rolling around on the asphalt. That was not smart. CJ ran over to our group. (CJ smoked a lot and he NEVER ran, anytime or anywhere unless it was playing ball.) He screamed at the top of his lungs.

"YOU MOTHAFUCKERS OWE ME," he screamed. "YOU OWE ME. EVERY LAST SWINGING DICK HERE OWES ME," he added as he got in each one of our faces. "ALL OF YOU. YOU THINK THAT'S FUNNY? YOU'LL ALL BE ON THAT FUCKING HILL IN YOUR GEAR AND MASKED UP, AFTER CLASS," he shouted. "THEN WE'LL SEE HOW FUNNY IT IS, DUMB ASSES," he spat as he turned and walked away. "I'LL SHOW YOU FUNNY," he added.

I'd never done pushups with fifty pounds of gear on, breathing from an SCBA, but how bad could it be? GOD, IT WAS BAD. It took us twenty minutes to do twenty pushups. Tomorrow was our first day of practical testing and the *real* shit was about to hit the fan. Daniels was a no-show and all seven women were dismissed from class early. Fire school was about to become a media circus.

The Terminators

It was made very clear to us what had happened the day after the dismissals. The chief of training (Halston) addressed us right after roll call. He told us that Daniels had quit and the women were terminated for "failing to complete evolution testing requirements within the time allotted by NFPA 1001 standards." All seven women had failed their first testing station and that was it, they were axed (no pun intended).

It was the top news story that evening and we all got some TV time, too. Camera crews were there the next morning and filmed Jimmy and I raising the flags. The county council had to get their hands in the shit, too. One female councilpersons was especially vocal. She had a lot of questions and all of them were answered. She had requested that the staff of the academy take her through each evolution. She attended class on one of our testing days and watched intently as we all passed our tests. She advised the chief of the department that she wanted to see if she could do it—"it" referring to an evolution, or two. She was seventy years old and this was going to be a hoot.

The following day, the entire county council was in attendance. We tried not to laugh at the old lady in turnout gear, as we were ordered to stand in formation. CJ was watching us like a hawk, especially me. Ever tried not to laugh, but the harder you tried, the harder it was not to (until you had tears in your eyes—then finally just lost it)? Guess where we were after class? Yep— pushups for the entire class (no gear this time and we had to do fifty). It was worth every stinking one. Amazingly, the old lady had finished two evolutions faster than any of the departed women. The staff didn't require her to wear an SCBA, which really wasn't fair. Adding thirty-five pounds to your back is going to slow you down and make a difference, I don't care who you are. Nevertheless, the women were not allowed back to class and Daniels had just had enough.

With practical testing complete, the final physical test was the timed run. NFPA 1001 required us to run one-and-a-half miles in eleven minutes or less. Of course, we were being tested for a three-mile run with the fastest mile-and-a-half counting as your test time.

Hammerjacks was my favorite club of all times. It was a rock club located in South Baltimore. I was a regular there and a couple of my buddies from Baltimore city went there, so I hung out with them. The women were hot there, too. I shouldn't have gone there the night before my run. Don't get ahead of me now. Monday was a beautiful morning for a run, unless you were me. I had a God-awful hangover and got to class just under the wire. I'm surprised I was on time and I felt like shit. There was no coffee this morning—it was ice water.

On your mark, get set, GO—and off I went, hating life, and running like I had lead boots on. The instructors were going to shout your time out as you finished the first mile-and-a-half, then you'd know if you had to run the next one faster. I was ready to puke as I neared the start-finish line for the first time.

"PRAYCHECK, TEN-FORTY-EIGHT," CJ shouted as I lumbered by.

"It's Praschak, sir," I returned in a failing voice.

"WHATEVER. YOU MADE IT, NOW KEEP RUNNING," he barked. I made it, but am I going to die? I was really struggling but I knew that once I got to the top of the hill for the second time, I'd be home free. I was really pushing myself to finish as I crested the hill and saw the finish line ahead. I ran with all I had and just wanted it to end.

Whenever we ran, we were told to keep moving after we finished and cool down gradually to avoid cramping. I crossed the finish line and immediately collapsed in the grass in front of the headquarters building. CJ handed his stopwatch and clipboard to another instructor and ran over to me. It was the second time I ever saw him run. He wasn't coming over to check on my well-being or congratulate me either.

"GET UP, GOD DAMMIT. DIDN'T YOU LEARN NOT TO STOP AFTER YOU RUN, DUMB ASS? YOU'RE GONNA CRAMP UP, THEN YOU'RE REALLY GONNA BE A WORTHLESS PIECE OF SHIT. GET THE FUCK UP, NOW, MISTER. IF I HAVE TO FILL OUT PAPERWORK ON YOUR SORRY ASS, YOU'RE GONNA OWE ME, NOW GET UP," he screamed, at the top of his lungs. I just lay there. What was he gonna do, kill me? It was too late for that, I was already dead, and he would have done me a favor, anyway. Jimmy had just finished his run and saw the festivities. He came to my rescue, helping me up off the grass and getting me moving.

"YOU BETTER HELP HIM UP. YOU'RE LUCKY YOU DON'T HAVE A FOOT IN YOUR ASS, BOY. GET OFF MY FUCKING GRASS AND HIT THE SHOWER, YOU MAGGOTS, BOTH OF YOU, AND PRAYCHECK, YOU OWE ME," he shouted.

"It's Praschak, sir," I mumbled, as I used Jimmy as a crutch.

"YOU'RE PUSHING IT, MISTER, NOW GET OUT OF MY SIGHT BEFORE I REALLY GET PISSED," CJ warned, as he returned to his post at the finish line. Get pissed? I thought he was gonna have a stroke, already. The funny part of the whole thing was, I ran my second mile-and-a-half, ten seconds faster than my first—10:38.

The hard part was over and I had passed all my physical tests with ease (well, except the run). That was my own dumb fault and I can't say I disagreed with a lot of CJ's opinions, at the time. With three weeks until graduation, the final phase of testing would be classroom, over the next two weeks. I knew I was home free and for the next two weeks, things would be more relaxed (relatively speaking). We'd still have roll call and PT in the morning, then classroom all day. We were up to five miles' running distance, and it seemed like a breeze. I didn't talk about the weight training we did until now because it still hurts to think about it.

The head instructor, Baynes, was a real health nut. He ran marathons and always ate something healthy, like bean sprout sandwiches (even though stories abounded about him eating a shit sandwich on a dare while he was a recruit). He was very fit these days, though not mentally. That must be why they picked him for this job. Prior to the start of the class, he had convinced the training staff to fund a first-ever weight training program. He bought cement, one-inch steel pipe, and had a painting company donate fifty empty one-gallon paint cans. Are you picturing this? The cans were filled with cement and the steel pipe inserted and allowed to dry. They were "Poor Man's Barbells." In the end, most of them weighed twenty-five pounds with a half-dozen weighing thirty-five, for the bigger guys in the class.

We started a weight program known as "Penn Reps" during the second week of class. It was a series of seven different lifts of ten reps that we had to do without ever letting the weights touch the ground (God forbid). When we finished the set, we'd end with ten pushups. We'd start with presses, flip our hands over and do curls, flip our hands again and do reverse curls. Then, over the head and behind the neck for hacks, followed by squats, back around for upright rows, ending with bent-over rows. Then we'd drop the weights and do pushups—ten of each was a full set. The first couple of weeks were a ball-buster for those of us that didn't lift regularly. I remember my arms burning, then turning into overcooked pasta in the beginning. While two squads were running, the other two would lift, then we'd switch. I dreaded the lifts more than the running. By the last weeks of class we were up to four-hundred and eighty lifts. That was six sets, counting the pushups as lifts—and they didn't hurt anymore.

One morning, near the final week, we had flexibility testing, and were measured. We compared our measurements to when we started the academy. I started with a thirty-eight inch chest, which was now forty-two. My neck went from fifteen-and-a-half to seventeen inches. I weighed 174 at the start and only dropped two pounds to 172. The difference was where the weight shifted because I was a lean, mean, firefighting machine now. The sad part was none of my original uniforms fit right. We were all going back to the quartermaster when class was over.

We finished classroom testing without losing anyone, although there were a couple that barely passed. I couldn't imagine that, because it was basic firefighting that most of us had before we got to this living hell. We had it drilled into our memories for sixteen weeks. The bottom line was, the men of the Anne Arundel County Fire Department Recruit Class 21 had been pushed to the limit by NFPA 1001 and all had made the grade. The last week was the best because it was roll call only. We were finished with PT and the days consisted of cleaning, painting, and general maintenance, preparing the grounds and buildings for Class 22. We even got a catered lunch of cold-cut trays and cold salads on the next to the last day. It was time for us to get our station assignments and I was having mixed emotions. I was graduating from hell and was actually going to miss the place. It was sad in some ways.

On the last day, we were to report directly to the academy classroom for roll call, in our Class C work uniform. There would be no more silly coveralls, spats, or yellow hardhats. We would receive our station assignments and be set free. Finally, the news came to me.

"PRAYCHECK."

"It's Praschak, sir," I added.

"WHATEVER. PARAMEDIC 26, 'A' SHIFT—GOOD LUCK," the instructor barked, with a chuckle added.

Paramedic 26 was the busiest medic unit in the county, in part because it was the closest one to the local hospital in North County. I was OK with that. *Nothing could be like Medic 16,* I thought. "A" shift was a good thing because I'd be working with Ken, and Cuz was on the same shift at Paramedic 5, so we'd be off on the same days. Finally, Chief Halston gave us his final words.

"Congratulations, gentlemen. I'd like to commend you all and extend to you a hearty job well done. You've proven that the tough NFPA 1001 Standards can be met with guts and hard work. I know we've been hard on you but that was our job. Our goal was to make you the top firefighters you are today. If we weren't tough, you'd have had a difficult time here. We're proud of you and will always remember Class 21 as the ones who set the standards. Graduation is Friday at the Glen Burnie High School Auditorium. Be there in your Class B uniform by1800 hours, and for the final time; Class 21…dismissed!"

"WOOOOOOHOOOOOOOOO!" It was a great day full of hugs, handshakes, joy, and sadness. My twenty-four classmates and I had become more than just "Recruit Class 21." We were family to each other and will remain family until we die.

Mom was better and I could tell that her and Dad were pretty excited to be coming here for graduation—so was I. I had a lot to be thankful for. The night of graduation, I got Chief Halston aside before the ceremony started.

"Uh, Chief?" I blubbered.

"Yeah, Mark," he replied.

"Can you do me a favor?" I asked timidly.

"Sure Bud, anything," he volunteered.

"Can you, PLEASE, pronounce my last name right, PLEASE?" I begged.

"Well, how's it pronounced?" he said in a puzzling voice.

Trying to keep my cool I said, with my teeth clenched, "It's Praschak…. Praschak…. PRAZ-CHECK. "

"Oh…well, why didn't you tell us before?" he said.

Shaking my head, I said, "I tried Chief, BELIEVE ME, I tried."

We lined the stage in our Class B uniforms—dress hats and badges, long-sleeved dress shirts, black ties, dress pants, and black dress shoes. Budget constraints had prevented the last five classes from being issued the Class A uniform, which included the traditional dress coat and trousers.

After the invocation we took our oath of office. Our names were called and, one-by-one, we marched up to the chief, gave him a crisp salute, accepted our certificates with a handshake, and joined our families. It was a great night. Mom was glowing and Dad was all smiles, too. It all felt so right. They knew that I had made one of my dreams come true and, by the way, the chief pronounced my name right.

Chapter 13
Perseverance

Paramedic 26 was supposed to be a "busy" unit because they ran 2,800 calls the previous year. Remember that Medic 16 ran twice that. Was I in heaven or not? I was NOT.

There were two differences between the units but, in essence, they were the same. Here, I worked a twenty-four-hour shift where the city was ten-hour days and fourteen-hour nights. Here, the average turn-around time for a call (turn-around meaning, from the time the call comes in until you get back to the station including transport and time at the hospital) was forty-five minutes. In the city, it was twenty to twenty-five. That's a big difference. I was about to learn what a twenty-four-hour ass-kicking felt like.

Déjà Vu...All Over Again

Alan and I really hit it off and he was one of the most awesome people I had ever met, like Cuz and Louie. Not only was Alan one of the smartest medics I'd ever met, he was cool. He was a former Marine that was assigned to the Presidential helicopter detail on "Marine One." This dude ironed his underwear. I'd never seen that before.

We really established a "partnership." He was married with children but always invited me to the house for birthday parties and cook-outs. It was the first time I ever had a "family" relationship with one of my partners, away from the firehouse. One shift, news came from the "Brick Shithouse" that we were getting a third person on our shift. It was Ron, the older, attitude problem, who I worked with at the Heights. Apparently, he had pissed someone off in the office and was being punished by being moved to 26. Wait a minute, who's getting punished here? Oh well, Alan and I just looked at each other and shook our heads when we got the news. I had worked with Ron for long enough to know that I would be the one calling the shots on calls and that was OK with me.

Waaaaaaaahhhhh…

"Medical Box 26-1, Paramedic 26, Ambulance 18 respond for a maternity, 201 Crain Court Circle, Apartment 3C." It was three in the morning and experience had taught me that this was probably gonna be the real thing. After all, there were no doctor offices opened at this hour. The apartments we were going to were borderline poverty-level and generated a couple hundred calls a year for us. Who knew what was in store? If it were a shit call, we'd send them to the hospital with Ambulance 18 and try to get back to sleep before we were wide awake and couldn't. Ambulance 18 was staffed by two vollies. The first thing Ron would do on any call was light a cigarette as soon as he got in the medic unit—before we even hit the street. It nauseated me because I was just starting to breathe, for God's sake. We arrived, grabbed our gear, and headed for the third floor.

I guess she's gonna be a big one, I thought to myself. Sure enough, she was at least 225, had broken her water, and was having contractions less than two minutes apart. It was her fifth child so the stage was set. I hurriedly did a quick visual check to make sure she wasn't crowning. MY GOD, THE CRACK OF HER ASS WAS FILTHY. I'm not talking, "a little shitty" either. It looked like she hadn't washed her ass in months. It was caked and I thought about poor little baby having to enter the world through this. It wasn't fair for him to start his "shitty" life this way. OK, that was wrong. The vollies on 18 weren't much better. One had a black Iron Maiden t-shirt on and the other, a gray work shirt, shirttail out, with dirty jeans. You could tell they were not professionals. We were taking her, regardless, and they would just help us carry her down the steps.

We got her into the medic unit and were on our way. I kept the portable radio with me, in the back of the unit. I told Ron that I would let him know if I needed him to stop on the way. We were about fifteen minutes from the hospital and I got the patient in the delivery position. I couldn't stop thinking about the poor little baby having to slide through her nasty ass when he delivered. I had to do something, so I got a large gauze pad (trauma pad) and opened a bottle of sterile water. I soaked the pad with water and wiped the woman's rear. ARE YOU KIDDING ME? I didn't make a dent in it and now I'm thinking, *Power washer and a putty knife.* This would be an all-night job and I didn't have time because on the next contraction, she crowned.

"STOPPPPPPPPPPPPPPPPPPPPPP!" I shouted into the portable radio. Ron brought us to a halt in the middle of Ritchie Highway. Fortunately, there was no traffic at this time of the morning. I had the baby's head out and suctioned his mouth, then nose. He was gonna be a big one. Ron walked to the back of the unit and just as he swung the door open. WHOOOOOOOOSHHHHH. The baby completely delivered with an explosive burst. A literal wave of clotted blood and amniotic fluid followed like a tsunami. Ron slammed the doors shut, just before the nasty wave hit him. Since we were on a slight uphill grade the "goo" pooled on the floor of the unit, at the bottom of the doors. I almost yacked. It's a damn good thing I was able to grab the baby's feet on his way out, otherwise, Ron would have been catching a screen pass.

I quickly wrapped the baby in a clean sheet and handed him to his mother. I was moving like lightning when I clamped and cut the umbilical cord. The smell was unbearable and Ron returned to the driver's seat. I told him to hold up for a minute as I opened the back doors and let the pool of pungent slime roll out onto the street. Unfortunately, a lot of it was laying on the back step. I figured it would be gone by the time we got to the hospital and they had a hose at the ER for calls just like this. It was Ron's mess, anyway, since he had been such a big help. We got back to the station at five with relief coming in two hours.

On the Move

Alan and I worked together for almost a year before he was promoted to lieutenant and reassigned to Paramedic 5. It was a sad day for me but I was happy for him. I had four months of probation to go before I could put in a transfer. I already had a plan and it was Paramedic 5 "A" shift, with Cuz and Alan. The shift after I got off probation, I got a five-percent pay increase and put my papers in. I worked at Paramedic 26 for six more months before my transfer was honored. A year-and-a-half there was enough.

With all good things come bad things. I was on the perfect shift, partner-wise but on the other hand, the station Captain, who happened to be on "A" shift, was an idiot. He was mentally unstable. I had heard stories of dumb shit that he had done, and that he hated paramedics.

Great, the one in charge is a hater, I thought. I worked with a lieutenant as a partner so I'd be safe, so I thought. There was a lot of thinking going on here, which was good. Station 5 had an engine, medic unit, battalion chief, EMS duty officer, and a reserve ladder truck stationed there. It was a newer station owned by the county—one of the three that were "volly-free." It was nice and it was a union station. The goofy captain was on the board of the local firefighters union. I was a member of the union in the city and simply transferred my membership to the county. I wasn't very active at first but would be in a few years.

We'd take the engine and medic unit to the grocery store to shop for lunch and dinner, usually in the morning after our station duties were done. The unstable captain would pull his pants up above his belly, turn his dress hat around backwards, turn his glasses upside down, and walk around the store like this. What an embarrassment. I'd walk out and sit in the medic unit and try to figure out what he was he trying to do. That was all the proof I needed to see that the stories about him were true.

I only worked at Paramedic 5 for two months before I was accepted into the upcoming paramedic class at the Community College. The county paid for us to go to college for a year to attain our National Paramedic Registry. I was going back to school and it was exciting.

The Next Step

I struggled with a couple of the college courses so I blamed the instructors. A couple weren't very dynamic and made learning difficult. Nonetheless, in June of 1987, I graduated from the certificate program. Mom, Dad, and my wife were all there. Wife, you ask? Shortly after graduating from the Fire Academy, I married a girl I had been dating for a couple of years. I never mentioned it because it was a mistake that only lasted nine months. You won't hear it mentioned again, until I remarry later on.

Once again, Mom and Dad glowed. Even though it was a one-year program, I shined with my cap and gown on stage. The next step would be taking the National Registry exam. I studied and practiced at the training academy, on my days off, with others that attended school with me. It was a grueling test. The written portion was given in modules and there were "prick" evaluators at the six practical stations. Some of the evaluators were local doctors and probably "haters," too.

I failed one module, by one question on the written test. I was able to retake that module again the same day and passed the second time around. I failed two of the six practical stations. One of them was a basic EMT skill station and the other was the trauma assessment station. The critique afterwards noted that I used "street skills" not "book skills." I ALWAYS THOUGHT YOU USED BOOK KNOWLEDGE TO PERFORM STREET SKILLS. I've been doing pretty well with that practice, so far. They noted that I didn't check for capillary refill on either of the patients.

Capillary refill is assessed by pinching the fingernail or pressing on the skin of a patient, and measuring how long it takes to get its color back. Normally, it occurs in a couple of seconds. In a person with lowered blood pressure due to uncontrolled bleeding, it takes longer. The longer it takes, the lower the pressure or the more of a bleed—CAPILLARY REFILL? The victim in the trauma station was bleeding to death. Do you think his capillary refill would be slow? OK, now I see how this game is played.

I had to wait two weeks before retaking the practical stations, then travel to a neighboring county to take it. They say, that gives us a chance to practice. Well, fuck practice. I took the re-examination two weeks later and passed. My application was processed and in December of 1987, I was officially licensed as a Nationally Registered Emergency Medical Technician-Paramedic. I finally made it to the top. I was officially a "Glitter Boy."

Back to Work

Once I returned to Paramedic 5, I was trained to act out-of-class. I got promoted to Firefighter 5 shortly after getting my EMT-P certification and that's one step below lieutenant. At this rank, I could be cleared to act out of class as a lieutenant. Alan trained me and in a matter of five shifts I worked my first shift as a supervisor. It was pretty cool. The paperwork sucked but I was calling a lot more shots and had more responsibility, especially on medical calls and, sometimes, the fireground.

Being cross-trained as firefighters and paramedics meant that we carried SCBA's (the air masks) and our turnout gear on the medic unit. Now and then we got to do firefighting as well as our medical routine. It was nice, unless you had a prick for a captain.

Waaaaaaaaaaaaahhh…

"Box 5-36, Engine 5, Engine 7, Prince Georges County Engine 39, Engine 28, Truck 28, Prince Georges County Truck 39, Paramedic 5, Battalion Chief 4, respond for a sign on fire on the roof of the Crofton Dry Cleaners, 1154

Crofton Centre, Route 3 and Davidsonville Road."

On box assignments, we'd follow the engine to the call, in case they needed to lay a hose line into the fire. If so, they'd stop at a hydrant, the aidman on the medic unit would grab the connection from the rear of the engine, and hook it up while the engine laid the hose to the scene. This prevented the engine crew from being a man short at the scene, if an initial attack was necessary.

We arrived to find that a welder had been doing work on the façade of the store and apparently started a fire on the roof. I geared up and helped the engine crew ladder the roof. My partner today, Charlie, stayed with the unit. I helped drag a hose line up the ladder, and then I climbed up with an axe and Halligan tool. It's a small tool about three feet long with a point and flat prying device on one end, and a pry bar on the other end. It's a pretty versatile tool when you need to tear shit up. It had started to rain. Frank, the firefighter on the engine, took the back off the sign with the Halligan as I used an axe to start chopping a lateral hole in the roof behind the sign. We needed to check for extension of the fire into the roof. Suddenly the captain shouts, "Hey, Frank, send Mark down here. He's got a call."

WHAT? I'M ON A CALL, RIGHT NOW. I threw the axe down and climbed down the ladder.

"You got a call," the prick said with a grin, as I walked past him. I bit my tongue because it wasn't worth it. I got to the unit and started taking my gear off.

"Where are we going, Charlie?" I asked my mate.

"Fuckin' nursing home," he replied. It was lunchtime, so it was a guaranteed shit call because the nursing home staff wanted to eat lunch. If I had a dollar for every time I went to a doctor's office or nursing home at lunchtime, I'd take a nice vacation to the islands. If I had a dollar for every legit call they generated, I'd be poor. They are, by far, the worst 911 abusers of all. I thought we were on the same team. I stowed my gear, got a towel, and tried to dry off a little before we left.

Sure as hell, it was a shit call at the nursing home. As we returned to the station, after the call, I said, "It'll be a cold day in hell when I gear up for that fucker again. If he wants my help, he better give me an order 'cause I'll sit my ass right here in this unit till he does." I kept my word, too. We had many more calls together. I never geared up and he never called for me. That was fine with me.

One day, we were getting ready for the annual station inspection. The paramedics' tasks were to clean the offices. As I walked into the bunkroom I found Pugsly, the firefighter for that day (Frank was off), tearing down the vacuum cleaner on a newspaper he had spread out on the bunkroom floor.

"What's up, Pugs, rug sucker broke?" I inquired.

"NO, the captain told me to tear it down and clean it,' he replied, with a bite.

"What? That's stupid. As soon as you fire it up, it's gonna be dirty again," I returned. He just looked at me with a no-shit-Sherlock kind of look. I shook my head and walked into the bathroom. I found Vern, the older engineman on our shift, on the bathroom floor. He was on his hands and knees, scrubbing the floor tile grout with a toothbrush. Am I working in an insane asylum, here? This is like watching a bad movie. It was rare that I wished for a call, so I could get out of the station. This was one of those times.

Waaaaaaaaaahh…

"Medical Box 7-14, Engine and Ambulance 7, Paramedic 5 respond for a child struck by an automobile, 2554 Marlton Way, cross street, Tilghman Drive." The dispatcher called. I didn't realize it at the time, but I was about to learn a hard lesson on this call.

Don't Get Close…EVER

Engine 7 arrived at the scene first. Within seconds, the radio blared, advising us to expedite. It wasn't a good feeling and when we arrived we could immediately see a circus of activity—cops, neighbors, rescue workers—it was pandemonium. Tom and I hustled through the crowd and found the crew from 7 holding down a nine-year-old girl that was lying in the street about ten feet behind a car. We were told that the car ran completely over her. She was crying and combative, and both of her forearms had open fractures, so she was difficult to manage.

Before we could do anything, we had to stabilize her arms and restrain her. I had the police move the bystanders back and it was obvious that the crew from 7 was a little overwhelmed by the whole situation. I quickly splinted and wrapped the little girl's right wrist and arm while my partner, Tom, did the other. I cut her shirt off. She had a black mark that looked like grease on her right chest, which was symmetrical, and she was breathing rapidly. The officer from Engine 7 had called for a med-evac prior to our arrival. The girl needed to go, and go fast.

Out of nowhere, a man ran up behind me and pulled me away from the victim. He got down on his knees and was trying to hug the girl. I got an arm lock on him and pried him away where a police officer took over. Damn, I've got shit to do here and I certainly don't have time for any interruptions. I finally finished my secondary survey of the girl.

Aside from the open fractures and possible chest injury, everything else appeared normal. Her heart rate was fast and her blood pressure was normal. It was a hot summer day so we wanted to get her into the unit and start an IV where it was cooler and quieter. The helicopter was fifteen minutes out. Seven stabilized her neck when they first arrived, and we finished securing her to the backboard when, the man appears out of the crowd again. We saw him coming this time. A firefighter from 7 and myself each grabbed his arms as he cried, "MY BABY, MY BABY!" trying to fight us off.

"Will you get this guy outta here," I yelled at the cop, that had taken him away previously. The cop and firefighter dragged the grieving father off. I felt bad for him but needed to do my job. Normally we'd let family members say goodbye to their loved ones before we left for the hospital or before we loaded them into the helicopter. This was not one of those times. Just as we lifted the backboard up and lowered it onto the stretcher, we got some bad news.

"Trooper 2 had to abort—thunderstorms coming this way," the lieutenant advised us. SHIT. The clouds were off to the west and that was the direction that the helicopter was coming from, as well.

"OK, LET'S ROLL," I ordered, as we wheeled the stretcher towards the unit. It just seems that, when things go South, they go there fast. The plan had changed now that the chopper had to abort their mission. Any time med-evac was grounded due to weather—patients would have to be transported by land.

Being in the metro Baltimore area made for long trips unless you were working on units up north, which were relatively close to Baltimore and a half-dozen specialty centers. South county units could make the trip by land to D.C. quicker than to Baltimore. We were in the middle today and the choice was Baltimore's, Johns Hopkins Pediatric Trauma Center, about thirty-five or forty minutes north.

Just as we were loading the stretcher into the unit I noticed a change in the little girl's mental status. She was not acting the same and after immobilizing her on the board, she struggled less but was still crying for her dad. She was quieter now and her eyes had a distant look, like a gaze. SHE WAS CRASHING ON US.

Tom and I quickly jumped in the unit. A firefighter from 7 would drive us to the hospital and was already in the driver's seat.

"ANNE ARUNDEL," I shouted to him, through the sliding front window.

"Anne Arundel?" he questioned.

"FUCKIN', GO. ANNE ARUNDEL, NOW DRIVE!" I ordered. Anne Arundel General Hospital, in Annapolis, was the closest. We had no time to travel farther than that. She needed advanced care (more than we could provide) now. As we sped off, I got on the portable radio and advised the lieutenant from 7 to make notifications to the family and police that we had changed our destination from Baltimore to Annapolis.

We raced toward US Route 50, the main line to Annapolis. Once on it, we'd make good time. Tom was in the "squad seat" at the girl's head and I sat on the bench seat next to her. She needed a lot of care quickly. As Tom monitored her breathing, which had slowed significantly, I hooked her up to the heart monitor. Her heart rate had slowed, too. Tom set up an IV bag as I grabbed the "start kit." I straddled the girl, on the stretcher, looking for a suitable site for the IV. I was hoping for a nice antecubital vein, which is the large one in your elbow joint. We could get more fluid on board with that one. Since her blood pressure was obviously dropping, the vein was flat, but I felt it. We rocked and rolled around turns, siren blaring. Tom had started using a bag-valve mask on the girl to increase her oxygen level. She hadn't stopped breathing but we needed to try to increase her effort. I had to balance myself on the stretcher and almost rolled onto the floor on a couple of occasions. This was what was known as "stretcher surfing," in our business, and it wasn't much fun.

Looking out the window of the unit, I could tell where we were. I needed a straight piece of roadway before I attempted the IV. It would probably be the only shot I'd have. We made the turn onto 50 and as soon as we got straightened out on the big road, I took my best shot. Like I said, earlier, this was my skill and I NAILED IT. I had a fair blood return, or flash, into the angiocath (needle). I got the fluid line connected and opened it up, wide open. The Ringer's Lactate solution was the only lifeline this fragile little girl had now. I felt good and sick at the same time.

It became obvious that the black mark on her chest was a tire mark and the car had actually run over her chest. Kids' bones are so pliable at this age, her chest looked normal in shape but the underlying injuries would prove to be deadly. My mind drifted to her dad and his attempts to get to his little girl. Did he know, by some Heavenly Power, that she was going to die? I heard her cries for him in the distance. They were silent now.

"MARK, SHE'S CODING," Tom shouted, and I snapped out of my momentary trance. The little girl had gone into cardiac arrest. My heart and hopes sank as I started one-handed chest compressions on her. I held on to the grab bar, located on the ceiling over the stretcher, with my free hand. I looked out the rear windows and noticed that the storm that had grounded our helicopter had caught up to us and it was pouring rain. Our driver had no choice but to slow down. I couldn't even see traffic behind us, it was raining so hard. Just then, a flash of lightning and a clap of thunder. Had the gods had come for her?

Tom was bagging her and I stopped CPR long enough to put the defibrillation pads on her chest and charge the defibrillator. She was dying and there wasn't much we could do about it. It was a cold and helpless feeling. Should we stop and get the driver to help us and wait for another unit to arrive with a driver, or should we keep going and get to the hospital as soon as possible? We kept going. "WHEEEEEEE...BEEEEP." The defib was ready.

"CLEAR," I shouted. ZAPPPP... Her little body was jolted. I delivered two more shocks, then continued compressions. I only stopped compressions long enough to do short tasks. I'd pump and get the drugs out, then pump, open the boxes, and set them up. I finally cleaned the injection port with an alcohol swab and pushed the medications—it's what I had to do without an extra set of hands. Tom was doing the same as he prepared to intubate the girl. As NREMT-P's we were trained to do direct laryngoscopy or endotracheal intubation.

Basically, we put a breathing tube directly into the windpipe of the patient. It was a skill that took talent and practice. No two people's anatomy is the same and kids and babies were even more difficult. We actually practiced on sedated cats while we were in our clinical training. A full-grown cat's airway is close to the same size as a newborn's. I thought it was cool but the PETA protesters didn't think so. They were always camping out in front of the hospital.

Tom short-tasked, as I did, and got the tube in successfully. We were doing all we could do but nothing changed. Tom had instructed the driver to call Communications, on the radio, and have them advise the hospital that were ten minutes out with a pediatric arrest, so they'd be ready for us.

Anne Arundel General was my favorite local hospital. The staff was awesome and we worked well as a team. It was the only staff I'd party with when we were off duty. We laughed together and cried together and that made us "family." This call would be no different. We arrived at the loading ramp at the ER. A doctor, nurse, and tech met us outside. As we wheeled the stretcher in, I gave a report to the doctor. He listened intently because he knew it would be a lot of info in a little time. If he had a question he'd stop me.

"Nine year old, no history, struck by car. We think the black mark on her chest is a tire mark. We thought it was grease, at first. She's got bilateral compound fractures above both wrists and her vitals were good, initially. She arrested on the way—coarse v-fib. We shocked her three times without change. It's a four-and-a-half tube and her airway's good—chest rise's equal with good sounds bilaterally. The IV's an eighteen and she's had about fifteen-hundred cc's of fluid, and three amps of epi. She's got a big bleed somewhere, Doc," I reported.

"Great—nice job," the doctor returned. Tom and I moved the backboard from the stretcher to the ER bed. The staff took over and we emerged from behind the privacy panels that had been put up. We had done all we could do and we knew that the outcome would not be good. I tried to prepare myself for the moment the room got quiet and the staff would come out, one by one. We'd look at each other and try not to cry. Emotionally, it was one of the toughest things to do. It was tougher than any fire school evolution, or refraining from kicking someone's ass.

The family arrived and was quickly escorted down the hallway to the "Grieving Room." It was a room that resembled a "gathering room" in a funeral home, I always thought. It had nice plush chairs, soft lighting, silk flowers, and a picture of Christ on the wall. The hospital's resident clergyman arrived shortly after the family. It was almost over, now.

The moment that we had dreaded finally arrived. The doctor was always the first one out because he had other patients to see. The nurses would follow, shortly thereafter. I felt bad and my heart hurt. I stopped what I was doing and thought about the events that had just occurred. It may seem to you that this all took a long time but, actually, it was a little more than an hour from the time we received the call. A nurse and a tech would clean the little girl up, remove the tube and IV, and prepare her to be seen by her family. After a few minutes, the attending nurse walked to the grieving room and stuck her head in. This, too, would a difficult thing for all of us to hear—saying goodbye.

Even though the door would be closed we could hear them. They'd emerge and you'd try not to cry with them. Then they'd return to the grieving room. I still couldn't help but think about her dad, at the scene. I sobbed as I rested my face in my hands, leaning on the stretcher. Gail, an attending nurse, saw me. She came over and put her arm around me, knowing that I needed some relief. It only made me cry more.

"It's OK. You guys did the best you could. We know that," she said softly.

I know—thanks," I sobbed. I was having trouble dealing with this and started feeling guilty about depriving a man from the last moments of his little girl's life. I walked away from Gail and down the hallway and opened the door to the grieving room. The father turned around and looked at me. I looked him in the eye and said, "I'm sorry, I'm SO sorry." He approached me and we embraced in a hug as though we were family members. We both cried out loud, in each other's arms. I kept repeating myself again and again…."I'm sorry." He said that he understood, that I was doing what I had to do. I felt so bad about it though. I told him that I had to leave, as Gail came into the room and walked me out of the ER to the medic unit. I sat on the back step, trying to gather myself. I was emotionally spent and felt like I could lay down somewhere and sleep for days. Gail had called the EMS duty officer because she knew that I needed some "extra help." By the time the duty officer arrived, I was better. At least I had stopped crying but I looked like hell. He knew that my shift was over and had already gotten someone to come in and finish the shift for me. The department didn't have an official Crisis Intervention team at the time. He ordered me to call Alan and talk with him as soon as I got home, but I didn't. I called Cuz instead. Alan wouldn't put a foot in my ass but Cuz would. I knew that I had made a big mistake going into that room.

This profession is full of life lessons. When you're "young and dumb," you have to learn. I learned a good one here and realize, now, how so many people burn out—they let themselves. I had to "reprogram" myself, I thought. I had to do what I could, AND WALK AWAY. I couldn't let myself get emotionally involved, WITH ANYONE OR ANYTHING, like Cuz had mentioned in his analogy—especially dead or dying kids. It was tough enough to work on them. As I said before, people would call us "calloused." Maybe some people that do this job are, but not me because my heart is too big. I needed to "reprogram" and Cuz was just the man to do it, like he had so many times before.

I saw Alan the next shift. Remember, the fire department is like one, big family, and news travels fast—especially if it's bad news.

"You alright?" he inquired, giving me a stern look.

"Yeah. I won't do THAT shit again," I replied, as I looked down at the floor. Al's shift was over and he was heading home. He just smiled and nodded his head as he threw his overnight bag over his shoulder and pushed his way out the door. He knew I had just cleared another hurdle.

Chapter 14
A Higher Power

If you don't believe in a Higher Power, don't even think about a profession in the Emergency Services. Trust me, it will make a believer out of you. Alan experienced a miracle, personally.

One day, after coming home from work, he got the kids off to school and the wife off to work, then went to work on his house. He was working from a ladder on the side of his house and somehow fell, landing awkwardly, and injuring his back.

His cries for help went unanswered because the neighbors were either at work or inside. It took him hours just to roll over and drag himself inside, using only his arms. Miraculously, he was able to get to a phone and call for help. When Engine and Paramedic 26 arrived they immediately summoned a med-evac.

Alan was at Shock Trauma for a week before being released. He had fractured vertebrae in his mid-lower back. His career as a field provider was over. He'd never have the ability to lift anything heavy again. I was offered a long-term acting position (more than five shifts) until they could permanently replace him. It was a great loss for the department and I had big shoes to fill. Was I up for it? I was going to try because I had his spirit. Semper Fi, bro.

Believe

Tom was Cuz's partner on "B" shift and we had worked together in the past when one of us was working overtime. Tom was a transplant from Ocean City. He had been in one of the first EMT-P classes at the college while he worked for Ocean City EMS. I always called him Beach Boy, because of his bleached blond hair. He was a great provider and we always worked well together. He was one of the only people I ever worked with that pronounced my name properly. You know I liked him.

120

One morning, Tom was doing the morning PM check (preventive maintenance) on the unit while I was mired in paperwork, and answering phone calls in the office. This check was performed every morning to make sure you were ready for whatever John Q. Public was going to toss at you that shift. Some of our coworkers were pretty lame when it came to restocking equipment and supplies that they had used on their shift. You'd better check everything when you followed a select few or you'd get caught with your pants down. Some would be so fatigued from getting hammered with calls and being up all night, you couldn't blame them. Some were just like that normally.

Waaaaaaaaaaaaahhh...

"Medical Box 7-14, Engine 7, Paramedic 5 respond for an injured person, eye injury, at the E. A. Grason Concrete Company, 2201 Cronson Boulevard, cross street Route 3." Seven's ambulance was already out on a call so we were the only medical unit dispatched. We followed Engine 7 into the scene, pulled up to the scalehouse of the plant, and met a worker that directed us to the patient. It was a hot day and the plant roads were dirt, which made for a lot of dust. We followed well behind the engine, so we could see. The call took us into a field where cement mixers washed out the remnants of their previous loads. There was a large above-ground fuel tank nearby. A man standing outside a company truck waved us down.

I was driving the day-half of the shift (Tom would drive tonight). The man ran up to Tom as we got out of the unit.

"My boy's fucked up. His eye is hanging out," he exclaimed.

"What happened?" Tom inquired, as he got the trauma bag out of the compartment. A firefighter from 7 was helping me get a backboard and the spine kit loaded onto the stretcher. We rolled the stretcher over to the passenger side of the work truck. The uninjured man explained that the concrete mixer drivers used the fuel tank. It was filled with diesel fuel and pressurized daily so they could spray diesel fuel onto the concrete chutes of their trucks to keep the concrete from sticking when they got to their pour. There was no electric service into the field so they would come out and pump air into the tank every morning. Apparently, they over-pressurized it today. It was a 500-gallon tank, which means it stood about seven or eight feet high, to the top. There was an air valve on top and, I'm guessing, a two-and-a-half inch steel plug. The plug had blown out and struck the younger man in the face.

"Holy shit," I said softly, as Tom and I gazed at this guy. His left eye socket (orbit) was smashed flat and his eye was dangling out about two inches. It was still attached by muscles and nerves and was, amazingly, intact and appeared uninjured. It was weird. Because of sympathetic eye movement (which means when one eye moves, the other moves with it), it was moving around. It was gory, but pretty cool looking. I had never seen anything like it. When the plug blew out, it hit him perfectly, as to not injure the eye but wipe out the supporting, orbital bones. It was still a facial fracture, nonetheless, and stabilizing it was going to take some delicate maneuvers. We loaded the guy on the board and stretcher and put a cervical collar on him, as a precaution, then got him out of the dusty conditions.

The road was like baby powder from heavy truck traffic. The company water wagon that wets the road to keep the dust down, was at the other end of the plant. Tom took a sterile trauma pad and gently supported the protruding eyeball as I readied an IV bag of Ringer's Lactate with tubing. We'd flush the eye prior to covering it then use the remaining fluid for his IV. The guy was in big pain (as if you didn't know this). Lying him down probably increased the pressure on his injury but we had to do it. We pleaded with him to try not to move around. He begged for us to give him something for the pain.

County medic units carry morphine and Valium, but city units couldn't. They'd be hijacked. I assured the patient we'd do all we could. All engines, trucks, and squads had plastic water coolers on them, year-round. The enginemen filled them with ice and water each morning. They also had Dixie cups. I opened the side door of the unit.

"Jay, grab me a couple of cups, will ya'?" I requested. Jay was the engineman at 7 and one of the only guys still working that was in Recruit Class One—yep, the first one held in 1965. He was probably the best breakfast cook in the department (next to me). Jay chuckled as he trotted toward the engine. He knew what I was up to and, like me, lived for calls like this. Anything that was a challenge and not the normal shitty diaper from the nursing home or headache from the doctor's office, we loathed.

Tom and I were on the same track without saying a word to each other. He had already constructed a "donut" out of a roller bandage (Kling). Normally, there are "donuts" carried in the trauma bag, pre-made, but somebody had used them and not replaced them. Like I said, you gotta check everything. Donuts are used for eye injuries that aren't protruding. They're about an inch-and-a-half thick, so you can put them over the eye, and then bandage without having the gauze touch the eye. We would use this one to pad and extend the cup.

Because of his sympathetic eye movement, we would cover both of the patient's eyes. Tom carefully threaded the donut over the eye and held it in place against the patient's eye socket. There was minimal bleeding at the injured socket and the "donut" covered it perfectly. I taped the bottom of the cup to the it, and Tom finished by wrapping the whole works with a Kling to hold it in place. Sometimes, you sit back and marvel at the work you have just performed and Tom and I did just that. We looked at each other, smiled, and gave each other a "high five." It looked great.

Now, after an IV, we'd head towards Baltimore and the Wilmer Eye Clinic, also located at Johns Hopkins. The guy was not in life-threatening danger, so there was no need for med-evac. Wilmer is the greatest eye hospital in the world. Baltimore was blessed with Johns Hopkins and my late friend, Dr. R. Adams Cowley, founder of Shock Trauma and the "Father of Trauma Care" in this country, if not the world. If I already mentioned that, too bad, it's worth mentioning it again.

"C'mon man...you gotta give me somethin' for this pain," the patient insisted. Tom and I knew that our protocol prevented us from giving morphine to this guy because of his potential of a brain injury from the flying steel plug. Morphine would cause an increase in blood pressure and increase fluid pressure on the brain, possibly causing it to swell. I had an idea.

"OK, man, relax. I'm gonna fix you up with some morphine. Give me a minute," I claimed. Tom looked at me with a puzzled look, like "OK, what are you up to?" I held my finger up, like a magician might. Remember that the patient can't see me because his eyes are bandaged. I grabbed the IV start kit from the trauma bag. I got an eighteen-gauge angiocath ready. It's a big needle, but not the biggest we carried. It's used for rapid fluid infusion and pushing certain drugs quickly (the blood bank uses the next size bigger (sixteen) when you donate blood). Tom was ready with the IV line.

"OK, mud, you ready? You're gonna feel a little stick now so hold still. It's an IV that we can give you your medicine through, OK?"

"OK, Man. Can you hurry?" he requested. I gently made the puncture and he flinched.

"Good job, man. Hold still a second," I reinforced, as Tom handed me the IV line.

"OK, you ready? I'm gonna start giving you your medicine. It might take a couple of minutes, OK?" I said, holding back a chuckle.

I opened the IV line, wide open, so he could feel a flow of fluid. He immediately relaxed his shoulders. After letting the IV flow for a minute, I backed the flow device to KVO or TKO (keep vein open or to keep open). It slows the drip rate to one drop every five seconds or so and keeps the vein from clotting shut at the puncture site.

"How ya' doin', bud, did that help your pain?" I asked him.

"Good, man, good. Thanks, man," he said, in a relaxed voice. Tom, the firefighter from 7 (that was watching), and myself died, trying not to laugh. It reminded me of fire school and the old councilwoman in turnout gear. Once again, it was "high five" time.

The patient's pain would return, twice, on the way to the hospital. Tom simply relieved it by opening the IV wide open for a few seconds. Anyone that thinks "mind over matter" doesn't work doesn't know what they're talking about. We tell that story to this day.

Comfort and a Kind Word

Placebos aren't the only things that would help me in my plight to save the world. Paramedic 3 (Annapolis area) and Paramedic 5 had more nursing homes, assisted living facilities, and senior citizen communities in their first due area than any other units. Of course, in the 1980s, it was nursing homes only. Regardless, we had a lot of older customers and I learned something about getting old—IT SUCKED.

Old people just seem to get forgotten, whether it's by their families, society, or the government. I hated nursing homes. They seemed evil and I can't think of one that I'd send my family members to, let alone, want to be in myself. We used to call them, "God's Waiting Room" or the "Last Chance Motel." I'd always say, *"JUST SHOOT ME, BEFORE YOU SEND ME TO A PLACE LIKE THIS."* I usually said it as we wheeled the stretcher towards the next poor soul that lived in one. There were very few staff members at these places that enjoyed what they were doing, and it showed. Staff turnover rates were high and morale was low.

The ones that did care were great but few and far between. I think I met one, once. Anyway, it was sad and frustrating every time we would go to one. A patient, their family, insurance company, and Medicare paid BIG BUCKS for this? What a racket. I met a lot of doctors that fed off these people like fucking leeches. I hated them, too. They were nothing but quacks to me. The state had passed a DNR (Do Not Resuscitate) law for terminally ill or elderly patients. It allowed them or their families to make informed decisions and allow the patient's death, with dignity. It usually went hand in hand with hospice programs and was a grand idea.

Many patients, families, and those with power of attorney would complete the form but not have it signed by their primary physicians, which made it invalid. Why? If the physician signed the form, he'd lose a customer when that patient died. So he'd drag his feet and try to convince them it was a bad idea. When we would come along and find the patient in arrest or near death with an incomplete form, we'd have to attempt to resuscitate them or give them advanced care and try to save them. The families would go ballistic and we were stuck in the middle. This was a very common occurrence, believe it or not. We once had a call for a cardiac arrest at one of these facilities where the patient's doctor, who HAD signed the form was present and directing the staff while they did CPR. I checked the form to make sure it was legit and completed and walked out. I didn't want any part of that lawsuit.

The people in the nursing home business were lazy, too. If Granny farted at three o'clock in the morning, the staff would call 911 just to get rid of her—one less diaper to change. A lot of times their quack doctor would order her to be transported, over the phone, so he didn't have to get his sorry ass out of bed and come in to evaluate the situation. They'd make me get my sorry ass out of bed. I generated many complaints from these facilities and you know what? EVERY ONE WAS JUSTIFIED. I DIDN'T CARE. Regardless of the cost, those people deserved good care and most of the time—they didn't get any care at all.

Waaaaaaaaaaaahhhhh…

"Medical Box 5-16 Alpha, Paramedic 5 respond for trouble breathing, Kentmore Nursing Home, Room 180-B, Bravo, at Number 201 Seville Avenue, cross street Millersville Road." It was three in the morning and we were running with no engine and no ambulance. No sense in waking everybody up for a probable shit call. The firefighters used to hate getting up when we would get to the call, have a priority patient, and have to call for them to help us. That happened a lot, too. Another thing I always wondered about was why they had to give us the addresses of these places on every call? We went there so often, the medic unit had auto-pilot to the place. What did they think, we didn't know where it was?

We always loaded the whole shebang on the stretcher, when we went in there. It was a bitch to have to run down the hall, get on the slowest elevator ever made (they all had them), run to the unit, grab your intubation kit, get back on the "elevator from hell" (or was it to hell?), and run back down the hall. We didn't take the kit with us, one time, because the call was for a sick person. YEAH, A REALLY SICK PERSON. That happened to me once and never again. We'd never get used to the smell of these places, either. I used to say "They painted the walls with urine-based paint." We wouldn't notice the smell after five minutes but damn, open some windows or something.

Our patient, this morning, was a CHF patient (congestive heart failure). It's a terrible, debilitating condition and normally occurs in-patients that have had previous heart attacks and the resulting damage to the heart. Basically, the ol' pump is shot. It causes fluid build-up which normally starts in the ankles and lower legs and, if not treated, can lead to pulmonary edema (fluid in the lungs). This patient was not treated but, recall where he's living.

His lower legs looked like they were ready to burst. He sounded like a fish tank when he tried to breathe, which was another familiar sound to us. The sad thing is, a patient that has this much edema didn't get it in an hour or two. Even if the shift at the home started at twelve instead of eleven, someone should have, at least, picked up the edema in his legs, or listened to his lungs. My bet is, they never did a thing at shift change. They made sure he was breathing, if that. This happened all the time and I could write a separate book on the shit I've seen in nursing homes, but it makes me too angry. I'd need anger management before I got to Chapter 2.

Of course, the staff said they checked him "an hour ago"—their records showed that. It was always the same old, "an hour ago," bullshit story. Now they're insulting my intelligence and I'm getting more pissed. We called for the engine, for assistance, and started working on the poor old man. It would never fail but the staff always disappeared on calls like this—like clockwork. It would be rare for anyone to stay in the room with us, unless the call was legit. I remember a few that were. If the staff knew they had fucked up and knew we were on to them, they didn't want anymore questions from us. It was sickening to me and didn't make me fun to be around. I guess that's another reason they fled.

We would treat this patient, transport him to the hospital and, if he survived, he'd eventually be released and brought back to the home. Would we see him again? More than likely, because they were "frequent flyers." After a while, I'd get a call during the day, walk through the place, and have people calling me by name, like I was a fucking resident there. I'd see some of those old folks more than I see my own family.

"Hey, how ya' doin' today, Pop? Good? OK, uh-huh, alright, see ya' later," I'd say with a wave, as we rolled our stretcher, stacked with equipment, down the hallway. Then I'd think about how true that statement was.

A Touch of Class

Over the years, I grew fond of my old folks. I liked to think that I was one of their favorites. My parents were aging and so was I. Someday, God willing, I'll be a crotchety old man that will tell you like it is.

I found that a simple handshake or even holding hands, right from the beginning, worked miracles. It really did. I'd walk in and address them as "young man" or "young lady" and immediately give them a gentle handshake or a simple touch. I'd sit next to them, close, if possible and (if it wasn't obvious) ask them what was bothering them today. I could get a lot from that simple question and usually did.

A lot of times there were many complaints that went back months. Others were afraid to call for help, thinking that they were a bother to someone. These were patients that really needed our help. They'd sit around, without treatment, and get seriously ill. When they couldn't stand the pain or sickness anymore, or feared impending death, only then, would they call. Sometimes it proved deadly, too. If you were kind and gentle, yet professional, you could have your way with them. It was especially hard to get the "old man" to go, whose wife had called. She would be upset at him for not wanting to go and he would be mad at her for calling. Situations like that took patience and hard work. He didn't want to go but she knew he was getting sicker by the day. After all, she lived with him. I'd be in the middle trying to persuade him to go, sometimes giving him scary scenarios of what the outcome might be if he didn't. I had to be careful with that. Sometimes it would backfire and make things worse if you got things out of context. A lot of times, you weren't going to convince them to go, period.

127

The Admiral

I remember working a shift of overtime at Paramedic 3. It was winter, and cold and flu season was in high gear. Three had several seniors communities that had many retired Navy veterans residing in them. Annapolis is the home of the U.S. Naval Academy.

I went to a call for a sick person at one of the residences, on this evening. I arrived to find a grumpy old man in his nineties—mid-nineties, I think. He was not a pleasant person and he lived alone. His home care nurse had arrived this evening and, in her evaluation, found that the Admiral's temperature had risen to 102. She advised us that he had not been feeling well for a week and was taking over-the-counter medications without improvement. He really was a retired Admiral, too.

I was very nice to him, held out my hand, and introduced myself. He reluctantly shook my hand and growled something about "being fine" and "damn doctors." I explained to him that pneumonia was a bad thing, and was going around. I always told them something was going around but usually, they knew it was the truth because all their friends were sick, too. I told him that we all wanted him to get treated, come back home, and get better. He was cooperating but bitching the whole time and my mission was to be the nicest person he'd ever met.

We loaded him into the unit and took off for Anne Arundel General under routine conditions. The siren would only upset him more. After all, he had a fever. I tried making small talk and asked a simple question about his military background. Without another word from me, he started. I couldn't shut him up after that.

He told me that he had graduated from the Naval Academy in 1922 and was a Navy captain at the ripe old age of twenty-five. He was telling me story after story and some of them were comical. We were laughing and having a good old time. My partner, Mike, said he looked in the mirror to see who was back there with me. He thought I might have picked someone else up at the last traffic light. The Admiral and I had great time on the trip in.

When we arrived at the ER, he was jovial and very nice to the triage nurse. A couple of minutes later, I asked him if Mike could take a picture of him and I. He agreed without hesitation so I went to the unit and grabbed my digital camera. I have that picture on my website today. He was a special person I'll never forget—The Admiral. I wish I could remember his name.

Depression Is Depressing

I was amazed at the number of old folks I'd met that lived in nursing homes or alone, had family members in the area, and never saw them—hell, never even talked to them on the phone, for that matter. You want to know why old folks get depressed? Aside from having nagging illnesses or the effects of just getting old, they get lonely. I get depressed just thinking about it.

My parents and brother have lived in Ohio since I was eighteen. They moved there when my dad got a promotion in 1974. I only see them two or three times a year and call them at least once a month. It really bothers me that a "family" could abandon an elder that, sometimes, lived in the same zip code or on the same street. It doesn't compute because family, is family. You can never change that. The gods put us on this rock to take care of each other. For God's sake take care of YOUR OWN.

Holidays are the worst, especially Thanksgiving and Christmas. We would always seem to get a half dozen calls where we'd arrive, find nothing wrong with the patient, or they'd change their chief complaints two or three times, right before our eyes. It was sad because all they really wanted was someone to talk to, companionship, or at least someone to listen to what they had to say. They wanted to go to the hospital. It was like they were living in "solitary confinement" in their own homes. At least the nursing homes and the ER put up a freaking Christmas tree for them.

If you're reading this and have elderly family members that you haven't seen or called in the last month (at the most), YOU BETTER GET OFF YOUR DEAD ASSES AND VISIT OR AT LEAST GIVE THEM A CALL. It'll be too late when they're gone forever.

In 1985, patients who had bypass surgery had a life expectancy of seven years. Mom was healthy after her heart attack and lived for fifteen years before dying in her sleep on August 1, 2000. She was sixty-nine, and was happily married to my dad for forty-eight years. We had a small private service for her at the local funeral home in Cincinnati, where she rested. It took the department fourteen years, after my graduation, to issue me a Class "A" uniform. I wore it that day because she never got to see me wear it.

Chapter 15
Once a Grunt, Always a Grunt

Acting as a lieutenant on "A" shift for eight months was interesting but I was glad to get back to my regular routine when they finally filled Alan's vacancy. I enjoyed being a "grunt" paramedic, working in the "trench." Honestly, they could keep that lieutenant's job. It was a pain in the ass and when they said "shit rolls downhill" they were certainly right. It rolled from the Brick Shithouse down through the ranks, landing squarely on the lieutenants. It wasn't for me because I was self-motivated and worked hard. I didn't need a lot of supervision and I think that's why they wanted me to work with a lieutenant (so he didn't have to babysit and could get shit done).

The Burnouts

In my spare time I played for one of the fire department softball teams. We were called "The Burnouts" and I could end this section right now because the name says it all. We were the classic "drinking team with a softball problem."

I played rec baseball from the age of six, three years of high school baseball, and league softball for years. I considered myself average (with moments of "aboveaverageness"—that's a word I just made up). My team, on the other hand, was mostly "wannabe" big leaguers and players that the other fire department teams had rejected.

The bottom line was, we had fun, and we were fun to watch. We played in a county league one night a week and entered all the local fire department benefit tournaments, including the Detroit Firefighters Burn Center tournament. A "drinking team with a softball problem" on a six-day road trip, with a hundred fire department softball teams from across the country and Canada. I could write a book about the three times I made that journey, too. It wouldn't be a children's book, though.

We were practicing for Detroit in August of '88. Three of our department's teams had gathered at a local park for a scrimmage one evening. I was playing my normal position in left field. "The Plugs" were the opposing team and were at bat. The department had teams that came and went over the years. "The Plugs" were one the better of the teams. There were "The Geezers," consisting of the older guys in the department (like that wasn't obvious) and "The Fire Girls." (yes, girls—we called them "The Clams." Oh yeah, when two women were riding an EMS unit we referred to it as a "clambulance.")

A skinny engineman named Jimmy who played for The Plugs, came to bat. He didn't look like he could hit the ball far but I had chased one of his hits over my head before. I backed up about four steps. Sure enough, he crushed one my way. I didn't even look up, just took off running and I caught up to it. I looked up and was going to catch this one, I thought. The grass was pretty high and was likely due to be cut, but that didn't slow me down. Suddenly, like they say, "something went terribly wrong." My right foot came down on something in the grass while I was at top speed. I felt my right knee pop and, down I went. It was the worst pain I had ever felt in my life. I landed on my stomach, crying out in pain.

I laid there, glove off, grabbing the turf. In a matter of seconds my teammates, Paul and Smut, were at my side. I don't think they thought I was hurt as bad as I really was. They rolled me over onto my back. The pain immediately went away—completely. I had two fists full of sod. They pried my fingers open, threw the pieces of turf aside, and brushed my hands off.

"You alright, man?" Paul asked.

"FUCK NO, I'M NOT ALRIGHT. I blew my fucking knee," I sobbed. Terrible thoughts were going through my head. One of the first things I thought about was how long it had been since I had surgery. There was no question in my mind that it was in my future—then "What the hell did I step on?"

"C'mon, man. Try to stand up," Smut ordered. He was the player/coach.

"Alright, but I'm telling you, it's fucked up," I insisted. They hoisted me up and supported me under each of my arms. I was standing on my good leg and was still puzzled at how such terrible pain could disappear so quickly.

"Try to put some weight on it," Paul requested, as he lowered the lifting pressure under my right arm.

"FUCK," I shouted, as my knee buckled and the pain returned, shooting into my groin like a hot sword. I almost threw up on them.

"Alright, you're fucked up. C'mon," Smut admitted, as the two lowered me into a cradle lift.

WELL, NO SHIT, SHERLOCK. I KNEW THAT. They carried me off the field. There were no benches at this field so they lowered me onto a large cooler that was on the sideline.

"DON'T SIT HIM ON THE BEER!" came the cries from my compassionate teammates in the field. I just flipped them the bird—my brothers. Nice.

A lieutenant that had a take-home car with a fire department radio had already called for an ambulance. I told him to let somebody know I was calling in sick tomorrow, and he chuckled. The ambulance arrived and took me to the local ER at North Arundel Hospital. I had x-rays, a knee brace, crutches, a prescription, and a referral to an orthopedic surgeon, when they released me. My girlfriend, Sandy, picked me up and took me back to the field to retrieve my vehicle. It was dark by then and I wanted, so badly, to limp down to the field and find what it was that had I stepped on. Later, I thought—later. I didn't have a problem driving but it took me fifteen minutes to get in, and out of my Jeep.

Light Duty Sucks

I didn't make an appointment with the doctor that was recommended to me by the hospital. I called a doctor I had met while I worked in the city, the next day. He was the director of Sports Medicine at Union Memorial Hospital in Baltimore. He instructed me to get a copy of my x-rays and report to his "knees, shoulders, and elbows man" at 10:30. I did but the news was mostly bad, with a side order of good. After a joint test and a needle the size of a McDonald's straw jabbed under my kneecap (I screamed so loud my girlfriend's son ran off and was missing for an hour), the results were in. I had a third-degree ACL tear, which was a complete tear of my anterior cruciate ligament in my right knee. The good news was there was no meniscus (cartilage) damage. They said I was one of the very few that had one injury without the other. Am I supposed to feel good now? Surgery was scheduled in two weeks, but I had planned on going to Maine with Sandy and her son, and staying with her family at their place in Bar Harbor, for vacation. The doc said, "Fine, but no rock climbing or break dancing"—Mr. Funny Guy, and I was not in the mood. I needed a vacation, right now, anyway.

When I returned from vacation my surgery lasted five hours and I was in the hospital for five days. I ended up off duty and on crutches for two months before getting a walking brace. It was then that I was released by my doctor to return to work on light duty. Sandy's son, Paul, was eight years old, and about two weeks after my surgery, had a little league baseball game at the park where I got injured. I loved getting out of the house these days. Since I lived alone at the time, Sandy's parents had set up a roll-away bed in their dining room and taken me in until I was able to climb steps again (the apartment I lived in was on the second floor of a residence). Paul was playing on the field next to the scene of my injury so we had to walk across the grass in the vicinity of where I had gone down. I told them to go ahead of me because I was slow-moving on my crutches. The grass had been cut recently and I thought that now would be a good time to look for the cause of my injury (if it was still there). I searched for a few minutes until my forearms were aching with no luck. I hobbled towards Paul's playing field when I saw it—a six-inch diameter steel pipe driven into the ground, sticking up about three inches. It was barely visible in the freshly cut grass. *What the hell?* I thought. The pipe wasn't very easy for the groundskeepers to see either because it had a large gouge in it where the mower blade had hacked it. There was an identical piece of pipe about fifteen or twenty feet from the first one I found. It didn't protrude like the original one. I was perplexed. As I stared at the woods in thought, I saw soccer goal posts lying on the hill nearby, and then it clicked. The pipes were sleeves for the soccer goal posts. The goal posts were smaller in diameter and slid down into these sleeves. I was happy and pissed off at the same time. My lawyer was more than happy to hear from me the following day and the county, eventually, settled the lawsuit out of court.

Light duty was day work (non-physical, 8:30 until 4, with an hour lunch break) doing some kind of stupid shit somewhere in the Brick Shithouse. I got assigned to the Operations Division where I sat at the front desk and greeted brass, answered phones, and filled orders for forms that were requested from the field. I was a freaking "cabana boy" and I hated it. I was going to be on light duty for seven months. Will you shoot me, now? One afternoon, just before office hours were over, severe thunderstorms rolled through the area. That meant that all hell would break loose for the people working in the field. Communications always got hammered, too, and the supervisor from Communications burst into the operations office.

"Chief, I need Praycheck," the supervisor shouted towards the chief's open door, as he pointed at me.

"It's Praschak," I said, respectfully.

"Whatever. Follow me," he commanded. I had been in the radio room before and I thought it was pretty cool. We really got some strange calls from people. I knew this because I was usually on the other end of a few of them. The supervisor led me to a telephone and handed me a stack of dispatch cards. He instructed me on how to fill the card out, punch the time of call in, and what questions to ask. I already had a pretty good idea, having hung out there on my lunch breaks. The phone started ringing with call after call, for an hour-and-a-half straight. I took calls for everything from lightning strikes, to accidents, to flooded basements. Apparently, I did well because the next day I was reassigned to a light duty position in Communications.

On the Airwaves

I went through a week of training, on day work, before getting assigned to shift work in Communications. I was pretty content and the shift in Communications was two ten-hour days followed by two fourteen-hour nights, then four days off. That was awesome because I'd be home every day. I wished we had that shift in the field because most twenty-four-hour shifts in the field were killers, and you didn't see home.

I fell right into place as the "Lifeline" operator on my shift. Each shift had a paramedic assigned to it and the paramedic would take over the conversation after the initial medical call was taken, if any medical instruction was deemed necessary. I'd give instructions to the callers on how to stop bleeding, bandaging, burn care, and you name it.

The toughest thing was trying to instruct someone on how to do CPR over the phone. It was a challenge, and you know challenges and me. I loved it and I did well in there for six months. I got certified as an Emergency Medical Dispatcher and, more importantly, worked a ton of overtime. I really wanted to stay but when the day came to get released back into the field, I ran like the wind. I'd still get calls for overtime, which kept me on my game in the radio room.

Transfer Time, Again

After seven months' absence, a lot had happened at Station 5. Cuz had gotten transferred to Paramedic 10 (which was closer to his home) and I had a new partner. Ben was my new lieutenant. I had worked with him before and liked him. He was a new officer and still had a little of the by-the-book-thing going on. It seemed that anytime someone got promoted, they got paranoid into this everything-by-the-book mentality. I can understand having it until you proved worthy of the position but some guys (or girls) never let it go. They were miserable to work with, too.

I didn't have anything against Ben, but put my transfer in for Paramedic 10 as soon as I heard Cuz was there. Cuz was a short timer with only six years to go until retirement. I wanted to "absorb" as much of his brain as I could before he left. Ben and I had some tough calls in the following months that made our respect for each other grow.

Waaaaaaaaaahhhh...

"Medical Box 5-36, Engine and Paramedic 5, Ambulance 7 respond for a pedestrian struck, Route 3 and Route 424, near the McDonald's. " Route 3 was a two-lane divided highway—very divided. The median was wide enough to have shopping centers and businesses between the north and southbound lanes. In most places, you couldn't even see the opposite lane, for the trees or businesses.

It was about 9:30 on a weeknight when we received this call. I found myself habitually trying to picture the scene, while I was on the way, then going over protocols and procedures in my head before getting there. I was maturing into a true advanced life support provider. I didn't realize it then, but I do now.

Ben and I arrived, just ahead of the engine, and Ambulance 7 was right behind. We traveled south to get to the call and saw a cop with a flashlight signaling us in the northbound lane. The victim was struck and thrown, some fifty feet, into the median, and down a slight grade. Fortunately, it was mowed grass and not trees or a thicket.

We noticed a Harley parked on the left shoulder where the cop was. A big, late model Olds was stopped in front of the bike. The cop told us the story as we carried our gear down the hill. Andy, the engineman, set up quartz lights near the top of the grade to light the scene.

A girl was driving north on Route 3 and her boyfriend was following her on his motorcycle. Another vehicle, occupied by a male, pulled up next to the girl and started making advances and gestures at her, so she sped up—so did he. When she slowed down, he did the same. The biker boyfriend got pissed and passed both of them on the shoulder, then rode quickly ahead of them. He parked his motorcycle on the left shoulder just past an intersection and as the two cars approached, side by side, he stepped out in front of the male driver, motioning him to stop. The male driver proceeded to accelerate and RAN HIM OVER.

When I say "ran him over," I mean, he ran completely over top of him, causing him to tumble into the median after exiting the rear of the car. As Ben and I scampered down the hill, we could see it was going to be an asshole-deep-in-alligators kind of call. This guy was a ball of trauma and was still alive—barely.

The victim was a big, biker-looking dude, probably in his mid-thirties to forty, and over 250 pounds. There isn't much room under a car but he had just been under one. It made me wonder how he didn't get stuck. At any rate, it would be easier for me to describe the parts of his body that weren't broken, than the ones that were, it was that bad. It was one of the worst I had ever seen and med-evac was on the way. It was Trooper 1 who was twenty-five minutes out. We needed all of that, and then some, to get this guy stabilized.

This poor guy looked like a freaking pretzel. I'm sorry, but that's the best I can do right now. Andy and I struggled to get his limbs straightened out. He had a weak pulse, and severely labored breathing. Frank, the firefighter on the engine, started bagging him, trying to force air into his battered lungs. The victim's arms were limp and went by his sides easily but his legs were a different story. Ben was getting equipment on the patient and setting up for an IV (or two). Andy held the guy's belt while a pulled on his left ankle to try to get the leg close to inline. The crunching of bones sent chills down my spine. I looked at Andy and for a big, crazy, tough guy, that had been doing this twice as long as I had, he looked like shit. I thought he was gonna blow dinner, right there. The victim's jeans were a twisted mess. I used my rescue scissors to cut away at the fabric up to his groin. The twisted fabric was preventing us from moving his right leg. As I finished my task I noticed a large, round, white ball in the guy's groin.

"Is that his nuts?" Andy asked, in a shaken voice.

"NO, THAT'S THE HEAD OF HIS FEMUR. I DON'T HAVE TIME FOR A FUCKING ANATOMY CLASS HERE, JUST PULL!" I shouted. Andy was a short-tempered, liquor-drinking, crazy son-of-a-bitch. After shouting at him I wondered if he would get "liquored up" one day when he was off, and come looking for me. I pulled the victim's ankle and twisted his leg as hard is I could. Finally, with one last crunch, the leg moved and we had a chance of strapping him to the board.

Ben had the EKG fired up and the victim's heart was beating at a tachycardic (fast) rate. I was amazed it was beating at all and wondered how long could it last. Ben had one IV started in the man's right external jugular vein in his neck. It was the only place we could start one because of the trauma to his extremities. We heard the helicopter approaching and they would land on the scene. Engine 7 had traffic cones set up in the northbound lane which were, hopefully, not too close. Rotor wash from the chopper made for tough working conditions. We finished strapping the man to the board just as the flight medic approached us. Ben told me to handle the pass-on of info and handed me the patient status sheet, after he notified Trauma of their incoming patient. It would be quick and I had to speak loudly to the flight medic, over the chopper noise.

"This guy has to go, NOW! Male, forty, completely run over by a car. We found him right here and he's been unconscious throughout. He has multiple disfigured fractures to his arms and legs. He's got head trauma, unequal pupils, and you name it, bro. We've been assisting respirations with the bag and have no breath sounds on the right side. An EJ's running wide open through a 14. BP was 90/50 and we couldn't get the shock pants on him. Trauma's advised, their waiting for him."

"Need anything else?" I reported and asked.

"We can't go to Trauma, they're on fly-by." the medic said, lazily. Fly-by meant bypass, or that the trauma admitting area was full. It must have been a busy night for them and it happened a lot.

"WE JUST TALKED TO THEM ON THE RADIO, THEY SAID THEY'D ACCEPT HIM; THEY'RE WAITING FOR HIM," I hollered, as loud as I could.

"That's not what they told us," he continued.

"I'M NOT GONNA STAND HERE AND ARGUE WITH YOU WHILE THIS GUY TAKES A SHIT ON US. I DON'T CARE WHERE YOU TAKE HIM BUT GET HIM THERE NOW," I demanded, as I stuffed the stat sheet in his top pocket, and returned to the patient. He looked at me with an amazed look. State Police flight medics are State Troopers that are trained EMT-P's, just like us. I normally treated all law enforcement people with the highest respect. They'd always say "Man, I couldn't do your job." and

I'd always reply with the same. This particular one didn't deserve any respect.

We loaded the patient into the helicopter. The flight medic put his helmet on and climbed in as we slid the door shut.

"Don't ask me where they're taking him," I shouted to Ben, as we trotted away from the ascending bird.

"WHAT?" Ben shouted.

"That asshole wanted to stand there and argue about where he was taking him. I told him we had talked to Trauma. He said he wasn't taking him there, that they were on fly-by. I stuffed the stat sheet in his pocket and told him to get the fucking guy outta here," I claimed.

"That isn't going to look good on your resume," Ben said, with a laugh.

"FUCK IT, I DON'T CARE. The man was lying there, dying, and he wanted to argue about it, for Christ's sake," I said.

"I feel bad for whoever's gonna get that clusterfuck dumped on them," Ben added.

"I hope it bites that flight medic in the ass," I said. It really didn't matter because two hours after arriving at the Trauma Unit at Prince George's Hospital Center, the guy died. They never found the car that ran him down and the Maryland State Police had been served notice. I wasn't going to put up with any petty bullshit, ever again.

In a lot of cases, the State Police med-evac helicopters flew into places in the rural parts of the state that didn't have advanced life support units or arrived at the scene well before the ALS units would. They would be the primary ALS providers on a lot of these calls. Some of the flight medics thought that was the case wherever they flew. I have to admit Anne Arundel County has a top-notch EMS program and a great reputation for having some of the best providers in the state. I was proud to be a part of it. The EMT-P program at the community college was the first in the state and students would travel from all over the state, Pennsylvania, and Delaware, to attend the program. Basically, all we needed from the State Police was rapid transport. They hated that.

There was definitely a rivalry between the State Police and us. This run-in wasn't the first and wouldn't be the last. There was a story that went around the EMS Division about a certain pilot that flew Trooper 1. He had a metal trashcan in the hanger, near the chopper, with the words "Anne Arundel County" on it. Every time he got a call in Anne Arundel County, he'd kick the trashcan across the floor. I don't know if it was true, but I'm sure that that can had plenty of dents in it. It would be a shame if he broke a toe.

Ooops, Wrong Way

Ben and I were working on St. Patrick's Day and it was a long shift. This holiday and New Year's Eve were called "amateur nights." Most everyone we encountered on these holidays had overindulged in his or her alcohol and done something stupid, then they'd meet *us*. We had gotten a call for a crash in 7's area, after midnight. It was a shit call and the engine cancelled us before we got there. We were on our way back to the station, northbound on Route 3, just north of the spot where the biker had gotten struck. As we approached the McDonald's we noticed headlights coming towards us, south in the northbound lane. Ben was driving and pulled over on the right shoulder as this car zipped past us. We just looked at each other with amazement. Fortunately, it was late and there was no traffic. Ben hit the lights and siren, wheeled around and stomped on it. Hopefully, we could catch up to him and stop him before something bad happened. I radioed Communications, told them what we had observed and had them dispatch the police.

We caught up to the car about a mile down the road. By some miracle, we never passed another car heading north and the wrong-way driver hadn't either. Ben laid the high beams on him. A male in his twenties, drove the car. He was by himself and slowed to a stop on the left shoulder (which was on our right). Ben slowly approached the driver's side and I was a little behind him, approaching from the passenger side.

"How ya' doin'? Do you know you're driving in the wrong direction on this road?" Ben asked, from a safe distance.

"Oh, I'm shorry, Offisher," the driver slobbered. While Ben distracted the obviously impaired man, I reached in through the open passenger side window, shut the car off, and snatched the keys from the car's ignition, in lightning fashion. Game over, we win.

This guy was a freaking Vlasic pickle. He was so drunk he thought we were cops. We had him stay in the car as we stood nearby and awaited the arrival of the police. Whether this guy realized it later on, or not, he was lucky that he came across us. He'd have *really* been sorry if he had to meet us the other way.

All Things Happen for a Reason

Transfers were coming within a month and Ben and I had been working well together. Our medic unit was scheduled for regular maintenance, one shift, so we had to change over into a reserve ambulance. It didn't matter what department I worked for, change over was still a pain in the ass. Most of the time the unit we moved into needed more help than the one we were changing out of, due to it's age. It was a hot summer day and we had just returned from the shop, in the reserve unit.

Waaaaaaahhhh....

"Medical Box 7-27, Squad and Ambulance 7, Paramedic 5, respond for an auto accident, Route 424 and Rossback Road." I remember wishing we were in our first line unit as we pulled out the door. As we arrived on the scene, we saw the crew from Ambulance 7 attending a teenage girl in the back or their unit. She had failed to negotiate a slight bend in the road, ran off the shoulder, and struck an embankment. The damage to the car was minimal and she was only slightly injured.

I was the aidman today and climbed in the back of 7's unit to give her a quick assessment. She was a non-priority patient which meant that 7 would transport her to Anne Arundel General. Ambulance 7 left the scene and Ben and I walked back to our reserve gem that was parked on the shoulder behind them. As we got close we noticed that the headlights were dim and the revolving lights in the light bar on top were barely turning. There was a pool of antifreeze under the unit. Apparently, it had overheated, stalled out and the lights killed the batteries.

We called Communications, advised them we were out-of-service and requested a tow truck. A county police officer that was clearing the scene offered to give us a ride to the shop when the tow truck arrived so we gladly accepted. The tow truck arrived about a half an hour later and Ben and I got in the police car for our trip. Suddenly, we heard a call come over the police radio. Two kids were found floating in a swimming pool at a residence, about a mile down the road from us.

Our reserve unit was hooked up and the tow truck was pulling away. Without a word to each other, Ben and I jumped out of the police car and ran in front of the tow truck, waving frantically for the driver to stop. We grabbed the pediatric kit, airway kit, EKG monitor, oxygen, and trauma bag, and loaded it into the police car.

"YOU KNOW WHERE THIS IS?" Ben asked the cop.

"Yeah," he said calmly, as he smoked the tires of the police car. I called Communications on the portable radio and told them what we were doing. We were a minute away and would be there ten minutes before Engine and Paramedic 3, who were en route. I was scared to death because this cop was flying low.

He blasted into the driveway of the exclusive home, as we arrived. A woman was directing us to the rear of the house. Ben and I were loaded like pack mules as we scurried to the scene. The two boys, ages seven and four, were out of the water and lying, motionless, on the concrete deck next to one side of the pool. Ben went to one and I took the other. As we went to work, we shouted our findings to each other.

"I GOT A PULSE WITH AGONAL RESPIRATIONS," I shouted, as I inserted an oral airway and started rescue breathing for the seven-year-old.

"A PULSE AND NO RESPIRATIONS, HERE," Ben returned. The police officer came to us with the story. The unattended four-year-old had fallen into the pool. His seven-year-old brother found him, a short time later, and jumped in to help him—neither one could swim. Fortunately, a male resident had found them. He said the four-year-old was on the bottom and the seven-year-old was floating about five feet down. Did he get there in time? Time would tell.

Without extra hands and both of the kids having pulses, Ben and I were content with our actions, so far. We could hear 3 coming and Communications had advised them of what was happening. I'm sure they were hauling ass to begin with. I had called for a med-evac for the pair as soon as we saw what we had and I know that Three heard that. They were a welcome sight as they came around the corner from the front of the house.

Paramedic 3's crew split and one came to each of us. We now had the ability to get the rest of the job done. The helicopter arrived a short time later and landed in a cut field next to the residence. Both boys were intubated and loaded into the awaiting bird. A medic from 3 would ride along with them. Anytime a patient was intubated or there were multiple patients, one of us would fly along with the flight medic to assist. I had logged many flights thus far and was sure there would be many more. Both of the boys survived their near-drownings.

Ben and I got a visit from EMS Division Chief McDonald, a couple of shifts

141

later. We both received a letter of commendation for our actions that day. He had also nominated us for MIEMSS (Maryland Institute for Emergency Medical Services System) EMS Providers of the Year, but just having him sing our praises made me proud, and feel good. I didn't care about a letter or an award. He also told us that the television program, *Rescue 911*, was interested in airing a reenactment of the call. We never heard another word about it after that day. I guessed the residents and parents didn't want to relive the story. I can't say I blame them and, besides, I'm a "street medic," not an actor.

Ben and I worked our last shift together at Paramedic 5, about a month later. I had been there for a little more than three years and had done a lot of growing up, but it was time for a change of scenery. It was 1989 and Sandy and I were engaged.

Chapter 16
The "Little Jake"

Station 10 was located in the old, remodeled, Jacobsville Elementary School building. The county had built a new school across the street and turned the old school into a police station and firehouse. It made for an interesting mix. Jacobsville (10) was close to the Chesapeake Bay, Stoney Creek (which was the size of a small river), and had lots of water very close, so they ran a lot of water-related calls. Shortly after the city of Cleveland opened the newly constructed Jacobs Field (for the Indians) and called it "The Jake," we named Station 10, "The Little Jake."

I was working on "B" shift with Kevin, my friend from the volly medic unit that had gotten hired by the city. He had made it into the county the year before me, and had just been assigned to 10 after his promotion to lieutenant. I knew a couple of the other guys on my new shift from The Burnouts and the union. The station lieutenant on "B" shift was assigned to the truck. He seemed like a decent guy. Any officer was better than that goof at 5. Rob, from Paramedic 31 was working with Cuz on "A" shift. This was a good bunch and I felt very comfortable here. The station housed Truck 10, Tanker 10, Ambulance 10, Battalion Chief 2, and of course, Paramedic 10. It wasn't a big, new station, like 5. Things were a little tight in the small five-bay building—hey, it was home. I arrived in March and Sandy and I were married in May. With the help of her parents, we bought a house in Riviera Downs which was about twenty-five minutes from 10 and two miles from the Chesapeake Bay Bridge, near Annapolis.

Sandy and I called each other Potent Pete and Fertile Myrtle when she got pregnant a month after we were married. Sandy wasn't a big girl and, after six months, looked like she had a basketball under her dress. We figured it was a boy because he was all out in front like her son, Paul, was. I used to make fun of her and warn her about turning around quickly and knocking people down, pushing things off a table, or knocking lamps over, but she wasn't humored. Things were going well at 10 when the big day came.

The Best Day of My Life

I was off the day Sandy went into labor. She had stirred me at about 4:30 as she got out of bed. I figured she just had to pee so I dozed off. I can't sleep if the sun is up so, without provocation, got up at around 6:30. Sandy had just showered and was in the bathroom putting here makeup on. I walked in, gave her a kiss on the cheek, and pulled up in front of the toilet.

"You going somewhere?" I said, jokingly.

"Yep, and so are you. I'm in labor," she calmly said, as she flicked the makeup brush around her cheeks.

"WHAT," I exclaimed, as I missed the bowl and hit the raised seat.

"I broke my water at about 4:30," she continued.

"ARE YOU HAVING CONTRACTIONS?" I excitedly inquired.

"Yeah, but you've got time to take a shower," she said, matter-of-factly. I'm freaking out and she's as cool as an ice cube. I almost busted my ass trying to get my shorts off and get in the shower at the same time. She grabbed her makeup bag and headed for the bedroom.

"Relax, will ya'? I'm fine," she ordered, as she closed the door. RELAX? *Sure thing, Sandy,* I thought. By the time I got out of the shower and got dressed, her contractions had gotten closer, MUCH CLOSER. I must admit, she *was* ready. She had gotten Paul up and he was clinging to her as they stood near the door. I wouldn't say he was actually awake yet. Sandy had her little overnight bag packed and was patiently waiting for me. I stumbled down the steps and grabbed the bag. We had a fifteen-minute ride to downtown Annapolis and it was morning rush hour, so add at least five minutes to the trip. Five minutes, hell, they knew we were coming. Traffic was a bitch and every time Sandy had a contraction or we hit a bump, she'd raise her ass off the seat and I would clench my teeth. I didn't want to deliver my own on the shoulder of Route 50. To top it off, we had to wait in backed-up traffic, in town, while Engine 38 from the Annapolis Fire Department's, Taylor Avenue station, headed out on a call.

"NOT NOW GUYS," I shouted out loud, as the engine bounced across the intersection. Our fifteen-minute journey took twenty-five minutes. I pulled up in front of the ER at Anne Arundel General. Paramedic 35, from Annapolis, was backed into one bay and the other was open. I left my Jeep running with the flashers on and ran inside. I immediately saw Dane, the lieutenant from Paramedic 35, as I headed for the sliding doors with a wheelchair. I met Dane years ago when I sat in on one of Cuz's study sessions. I'm sure he could tell I was excited as I hesitated long enough to speak.

"DANE, CAN YOU PARK MY WIFE WHILE I TAKE MY JEEP UPSTAIRS?" I asked. Before I could take another step, he had me by the arm.

"Hold on, partner. I'll take her upstairs, you park the car," he said calmly. I just looked at him, dumbfounded.

"Oh yeah, that'll work, too," I said with a blush. We both helped Sandy out of the Jeep and Paul followed as Dane wheeled her towards the ER doors. I ran around the Jeep, jumped in, and parked in a spot along the curb that was reserved for cops and ambulances. I didn't care at this point—I wanted to be with my family. When I got upstairs, I asked Dane to let Hospital Security know that it was my vehicle.

Sandy was in labor for about ten hours and at 1440 hours on July 27, 1990, gave birth to Michael Ryan Praschak. He was seven pounds, thirteen ounces and twenty-one inches with light brown hair and blue eyes, like his mom. He looked like he just got off the beach, though (at least he got something from me—my dark skin). I hope he gets to keep his hair longer than I did. The nurses immediately crowned him "Beach Baby." It was, and will remain, the greatest day of my life.

A Different Place

Paramedic 10 was a different place for me. When people live near or on the water, their activities and environment are different than those that live inland. I experienced a lot of calls that proved that.

Waaaaaaahhhhh…

"Water Rescue Box 10-14, Truck 10, Squad 13, Fireboat 13, Boat 20, Engine 12, Paramedic 10, Ambulance 10, EMS 3, Battalion Chief 2, Special Ops 1, Dive/Rescue Unit respond for a drowning, at the end of White Rocks Road, cross street Fort Smallwood Road. "

This was the first drowning call where I was going to be the first one on the scene. It was nerve-racking. I was working with Kevin, and I always got on his case about driving too fast. Today, it didn't matter. We couldn't go fast enough.

Seconds count on all calls but especially water rescues. A man and woman met us as we arrived. We listened to their account as we emptied our pockets, put on our orange life vests and hurried to the beach. *I* was going in.

A teenage boy was wading, in waist-deep water, about a hundred yards offshore when he went under and never surfaced. Kevin would direct me, with hand signals, to where the swimmer was last seen by the witnesses. The male witness happened to have a boat hook with him. It was an aluminum pole with a plastic hook on the end that could reach about eight feet when fully extended. I took it from him and waded toward the site. I walked most of the way then the bottom suddenly dropped off beneath my feet. I could see Kevin pointing with outstretched arms in the direction he wanted me to go. I was floating now and started probing the bottom with the hook.

During rescue class, I had learned that the dive team would set up a grid pattern of searching. I didn't have their resources so I used landmarks on the opposite site of the creek to start my imaginary grid back and forth across the deepest part of the creek. I could see other units arriving and personnel filling the beach. After fifteen minutes, a small rescue boat came blazing into the creek. A firefighter was at the helm of the small, center console boat, with a diver accompanying him. The diver's name was Ross and was a member of my fire academy class. The boat pulled up to me, slowly.

I showed Ross the area that I had started searching as he donned his tank and mask. He splashed in next to me and went under. The Chesapeake Bay and most of its tributaries are known as brackish water, which is a mix of salt and fresh water. There is no visibility, anywhere. Unlike the crystal clear water you see divers in on TV, this water is nearly impossible to see in, even a foot in front of your mask. Ross surfaced and I guided him to where I had started. We started the process again. I paddled to the start point and dragged the hook across the bottom. There were some places I had to submerge my head, in order to touch the bottom. I had always been a good swimmer and didn't have much fear of the seas. It was a tough task with the life vest and uniform on.

Suddenly, I felt something. I tried to hook it and splashed 'water bombs' with my cupped, free hand (like I used to do as a kid) trying to get Ross to surface. He heard me and when he surfaced, twenty or so feet from me, I gave him the report. He dove right below me and I hoped he would find something. Time was ticking with the warm summer water because the colder the water, the better the chances of survival. You may recall the story of the kid in

146

Minnesota that fell through the ice and was revived after over an hour under the frigid water. The water today was over seventy degrees and it was getting late. Ross surfaced, blew his mouthpiece out, and said,

"It's just an old crab pot." DAMN. We searched on and it was quickly changing from a rescue operation to a recovery operation. Just then, Ross surfaced right in front of me. His eyes were the size of saucers.

"I GOT HIM," he gasped, as he spit his mouthpiece out. I frantically waved for the rescue boat. He approached as fast as he could without 'swamping' us. Ross and I lifted the lifeless body to the 'gunnel' of the boat where the firefighter dragged the body on board. THAT WAS ONE BIG FUCKING TEENAGER! He must have been six feet tall and over 200 pounds.

The firefighter helped Ross into the boat and I was next. They both pulled me in with a fury. I slammed onto the deck of the boat, scratching my right forearm on something. It was six inches long and barely bled, but it hurt like hell. Ross and I started CPR on the boy as we headed for land. Paramedic 12 had been dispatched to assist us because I was on the primary rescue team. They had set up *our* equipment on a dock next to the beach since their unit was about a half mile up the road, blocked out by other equipment. There was limited access to the beach with all the equipment that had arrived ahead of them.

We offloaded the victim at a pier closest to the beach and the medics from Twelve took over. The victim didn't respond but we had given it our all. It wasn't going to happen today without some kind of miracle. On average, it was a quick recovery but, in all probability, it was too late.

John, an EMT on Ambulance 10, wrapped my arm. It stung badly and the chief in command had ordered me to the hospital for treatment. The creek we were working in had been declared unsafe for swimming because of a sewage spill six months ago—NICE.

Paramedic 12 had arrived at the hospital ahead of us and I could hear the ER staff working on the victim as the guys from 10 rolled me past the acute care cubicle. They had put me in a wheelchair and were taking me in to be seen by a doctor. A short time later, a nurse scrubbed my wound with antiseptic, dressed it, and gave me a ten-day prescription for Keflex. I went home and slept for eight hours, straight. The young man didn't make it.

Burning Down the House

A couple of our chief officers were famous for burning things down in the name of safety. This particular night was a prime example.

Waaaaaaahhhh.......

"Box 10-14, Engine 13, Engine 20, Engine 12, Engine 30, Truck 10, Truck 23, Squad 13, Tanker 10, Paramedic 10, Battalion Chief 2, respond for a dwelling fire at 1163 Paradise Beach Road, cross street Bayside Beach Road."

Chief Price was the first one out the door. We followed the truck and the tanker trailed. As the chief arrived he reported fire showing from the front of the single story dwelling. When Thirteen's engine arrived, Kevin and I helped drag an inch and three-quarter line to the front door. Fire was blowing out of the picture window next to the front door and a live electric service wire was hanging low in front of it, arcing.

A volly from 13 was on the nozzle followed by Kevin and myself. We entered the front door low and advanced about five feet inside. Just then, the volly opened the nozzle. Was there a problem? We didn't see any fire yet so he was a what we called, a "smoke squirter."

"Shut it down and move, shut it down and move," we commanded. He shut the nozzle down and froze. Kevin and I knew we had to advance to the fire room and knock the fire down before it burned through the ceiling and into the attic. Kevin stood on his knees and physically dragged the volly off the nozzle. I followed suit and kept the kid moving past me. Now that we had the nozzle we could get things moving and the volly kept moving, right out the door, leaving us alone.

We crawled towards the glow, which was around the corner in the living room, dragging the hose line with us. Kevin encountered a piece of furniture and raised up to move it when two large boards crashed down on us. It wasn't a piece of furniture he had moved but a sawhorse that was supporting two or three, big, pieces of lumber. Apparently the house was being remodeled so that was a good indicator that there, probably, wouldn't be a rescue. The place was unoccupied. We were doing a quick-search as we moved in, anyway. We pushed the boards off of ourselves and moved into a short hallway that led to the entrance of the fire room. Just then someone crawled up behind me and shouted,

"EVAC, EVAC," their voice muffled by their facepiece.

"WHAT? TWO MINUTES, JUST GIVE US TWO MINUTES," I begged.

"(Chief) PRICE SAYS OUT, NOW," he returned. Shit, we were there. All we need was two minutes to knock it and three minutes to back out. I grabbed Kevin by the top of his air bottle and said,

"Price says we gotta go, bro." He made the same plea that I had, but I told him we had to get out. We backed out, dragging the hose line behind us. Once outside we ripped our masks off and stood there, looking at each other. Steam, literally, rolled from our heads as our heated bodies hit the cool, night air. Kevin looked over toward the command post where Price was standing.

"Asshole," he muttered, as we trudged toward the medic unit. The crew from Truck 10 had already chopped two holes in the roof for ventilation before the order to evacuate. Within twenty minutes, half the roof was burned off the place. We sat on the back step of the medic unit and watched the vollies from 13 bail water through the now-gaping roof. Eventually they'd drown it out.

"I should be a chief," Kevin exclaimed.

In Memory Of…

In the beginning, I said that names would be changed to protect identities. So far this has been true. Those, who departed this world prematurely are still those who are sorely missed, to this day. There's a special one I'd like to tell you about.

Johnny was a likeable young man, in his early thirties, that worked at Truck 10 on "A" shift. He had been in the department for about six years and lived a mile, or so, from the station. I always thought he was a good guy because he worked hard and loved his job. He'd bring his kids to the firehouse on occasion and seemed like a real family man. He was diagnosed with lymphoma about two years after I arrived at Paramedic 10.

I know that not being able to work was not easy for him. I know he missed the firehouse as much as we missed him. He was in, and out, of Johns Hopkins Hospital frequently. I'll never forget the *one* time I went to visit him. He was having a bone marrow transplant the next day, so he couldn't eat anything the day before. I walked into his room and the first thing I noticed was a picture of a roast beef sandwich that had been cut out of a Roy Rogers ad and taped to his IV bag. We laughed and I told him I hoped he didn't lose his willpower and try to take a bite out of the bag. I wish, now, that I visited him more than once because that was the last time I'd see him alive.

Having used all of his sick and annual leave, Johnny depended on *us* to work his spot on the truck for him. He had no problem getting relief because that's what family was all about. I had signed up to work a shift for him and I know it was a shift he would have loved to been on.

Truck 10 broke down on the shift prior to the one I was working for Johnny, and we had a reserve truck. It was a "bend-in-the-middle," or tractor-drawn type, with the tillerman in back, steering the trailer. I told the chief on "A" shift that I was working for John the next shift, and asked him if he had a problem with me "tillering." Chief Gene knew that I could handle it because he was the chief on my shift when I was at Paramedic 5. He knew that I had operated the reserve truck there during routine PM checks in the morning. He thanked me and said,

"No problem." I was excited and it would be a nice break from the medic unit, to boot.

There was a possibility that the first-line truck would be repaired and back by the next shift. I called the station the night before and they told me that they had the first line back and that I wouldn't have to tiller, instead, I was Acting Lieutenant. Cool—I'd get to talk on the radio and blow the siren. It was a little more involved than that and it was a shift to remember.

Waaaaaahhhh…

"Reduced Box 10-12, Engine 13, Truck 10, respond for an odor of smoke in a dwelling, no smoke or fire evident, at number 1005 Fairview Beach Road, cross street of Fort Smallwood Road."

A reduced box called for an engine and truck or squad, which ever was closest, and was usually struck for smaller fires like appliances, dryers, stoves, and the like. Had the caller noticed smoke or fire, a full box assignment would be dispatched, like the one in the previous story.

We got there and traced the odor to the fuse box in the aged dwelling. It still had the glass, screw in-type fuses, not circuit breakers. While I got info from the resident for my report, a box alarm was sounded for a fire at a nearby bowling alley in 33's area. Actually, it was right across the street from Thirty-Three so they'd get there quickly. The screaming started right away and apparently it was lit. They called for a second alarm as soon as they got there so we went in service quickly. Maybe we'd get in on the action if it went to more than two alarms.

"Fire Alarm to Truck 10."

"Truck 10," I answered.

"Transfer to the First Battalion—we'll advise which station. "

"Truck 10 copied, en route to the First," I stated. We were getting closer. About two minutes later we heard,

"Fire Alarm to Truck 10, disregard the transfer. Standby to copy the third alarm." YEAH, WE'RE GOING TO THE SHOW! We were the first due truck on the third alarm and we had just gotten on Route 100, which was a main line to the fire. We'd be there in eight minutes and could see the huge column of black smoke in the distance. She was lit, all right.

I called the chief in Command, as we approached the scene, to get an assignment. The chief was confused because we had gotten there ahead of the second alarm truck company. He told us to set up a ladder pipe operation on the street adjacent to the bowling alley, on the east side. The fire was already through the roof. We would hook two water supply lines from an engine, to the truck, fully extend the ladder (one hundred feet), and shoot a solid, two-and-a-half inch stream of water, over the businesses we were parked in front of, into the bowling alley on the backside. I was pumped up because some guys go through their entire careers, on a truck company, and never get to do this.

The firefighter on the truck that day, Curtis, was masked-up and started his climb upward. It was work climbing the ladder a hundred feet at a seventy-five- or eighty-degree angle and I knew he'd be winded by the time he got to the top. As soon as he got positioned we started flowing water. The flames were shooting upward of fifty to sixty feet and, now and then, smoke would envelop the end of our ladder. We'd always wear a mask up there, too.

Thirty or forty minutes later, Curtis called on the intercom and needed a break. It was my turn to go up to the pipe and Curtis used a two-foot length of rope with a metal hook on the end, called a rope hose tool, to secure the huge nozzle before he descended. By doing this, we didn't have to stop the flow of water while we changed crew. I hadn't been to the top of a ladder since fire school but was anxious to go as I started my climb.

I was breathing hard as I got to the top and locked the large hook on my safety belt (ladder belt) onto the second rung of the ladder. I untied the rope hose tool and now had control of the pipe. It had a two-foot-long bar on it, so I could move the pipe up or down to direct the stream. The stream of water sounded like a small jet engine as the water blasted out at 200 or so pounds per square inch. I directed the stream where the biggest concentration of fire was, occasionally having to hold my mask up to my face and crack my air valve open to breathe, when the smoke column came my way.

A large portion of the roof had collapsed and they had just struck the fifth alarm. Truck 21 from Baltimore city was to my right and Trucks 31 and our Truck 21 were on the street in front of us, to my left. Truck 33 was on the front side of the building and I could only see their ladder and stream. It was a wild view. There were five ladder pipes on three sides of a pretty big building. I remember wishing I had a video of it.

I got real thirsty after an hour and needed a break. Curtis and I would take turns for the next five hours before we finally got the fire out and were released. As I climbed off the turntable for the last time, I was greeted by the chief of the EMS division, Chief Timmons—my big boss. Big fires brought out all the brass.

"Lieutenant," he said calmly, with a grin.

"Chief," I replied, with the same grin.

"Nice job, son," he said, as he patted me on the shoulder and slowly walked away.

"Thanks, Chief," I returned, as I poured a cup of water over my head. There was a growing rivalry between the Suppression and EMS divisions and it wasn't a localized thing, it was nationwide. The mentality was, if you were a paramedic, you weren't as tough as a firefighter. Well, that was bullshit to me because that was part of my title and part of my job—firefighter paramedic. I went through the same ass-grinder that they did but they don't seem to remember that.

I think Chief Timmons was proud to see one of his boys getting the job done. He was one of the smartest fire department people I ever met and he was known nationwide, too. We were like his children and the paramedic program had always been his dream, which had come to life. I felt good. I've pissed on more fires than most of the 'haters' have seen, anyway. We had a total of ten calls that shift including the "big one."

Thanks, Johnny. You gave me something that I would only have once in my career. I miss you and won't ever forget you, bro.

Work Wife

I was happy for Cuz when he retired. The union had promised him a great deal and backed the election of the future county executive, that had promised him a great pension—promises, promises. Unfortunately politicians lie, regardless of their party affiliation. Cuz had locked in the deal and was going out with high expectations.

The now-elected county executive that had gotten elected by a short margin, thanks to a lot of hard work and campaigning support from our union members. We had a difference of opinions at contract time and he reneged on his promise. Cuz lost sixteen percent of his retirement, but had already committed to the deal. Once again, I learned from him. With guaranteed raises of at least two-percent per year, or the equivalent of the country's cost of living increase, he'd be back to even after eight years—typical political bullshit. "We love you and appreciate your years of service, but, FUCK YOU," basically. It always seemed to be a one-way street when it came to endorsing any candidate. I always had my guard up after they screwed my mentor.

Even though the county boned him, Cuz was happy to be away from the job. He told me that every time I saw him. The most important thing he told me was, that I had to hang in there and finish the trip and I always kept that in my mind. It was good advice and I thought about it often, especially when the administrative crap would get me down. I was halfway to retirement.

Kevin and I worked together for a year before he put his transfer in for the haz-mat unit at Station 23, as soon as he was allowed. When he left, my new lieutenant was a girl named Maddy. She was a cute little blonde with two kids and an alcoholic husband. She loved NASCAR, gambling, and spending money. She probably couldn't lift her own weight but she was sweet, job-smart, and fun to work with. We had worked with each other a few times before she got promoted and she knew I would be her "muscle" on the job, as I was. She always referred to herself as my "work wife." We established that early.

I loved her like a sister but, eventually, rumors had us sleeping together, on and off the job. It was never true. I had thought about it, but that was it. I never, in my entire career, dated or slept with a coworker (or nurse for that matter), let alone a married one, and NEVER thought of doing anything at work. I had seen other guys and girls mix work and relationships. Most of them failed and they were miserable when they had to work with each other or see each other at work. I couldn't handle the thought of it.

Maddy and I were happy doing our jobs and going our separate ways when the shift was over. We had some memorable calls, too.

Waaaaaaaahhhh........

"Medical Box 11-7, Engine 11, Paramedic 10 respond for a cardiac, 6675 Weldon Road cross street, Fort Smallwood Road."

There was nothing unusual about that dispatch. If I had a dollar for every cardiac-trouble breathing-diabetic-sick case-call I ever ran, I wouldn't have to write this book. Engine 11 arrived and advised us that the patient was a Priority One. Maddy pressed on the gas a little harder. When we got there we found a elderly man lying on the couch of a modest little home. He had, "the Look," and "the Look" was not good. It was a cold, clammy, "yukky" look. You can tell someone is really sick when they have it. You don't learn about it from books but you sure learn about it fast on the street. The Look, usually, made everyone move a little faster than normal, and when you've worked at the job long enough with the same people, they get to know your intentions from your body language, and eye contact. Your adrenaline pumps, your heart rate goes up, you breathe fast, and you move quickly, but you can't let the patient or family know. You had to keep cool or the whole place would go nuts. I've seen it happen before, and I used to tell my patients "Don't get excited unless you see me get excited," all the time. It was one of my catch phrases. I had a few of them and I worked hard at being cool on the outside while I was, at times, freaking on the inside. It took a lot of practice.

The captain from the engine had reported that the old guy, who was home alone, had low blood pressure and he had no pulse. He was lethargic and didn't flinch when I spoke loudly into his ear. His respirations were shallow and his eyes barely open. Maddy was hooking him up to the EKG monitor. We looked at each other when the screen lit as she turned it on. He was in ventricular tachycardia or v-tach. The majority of cardiac arrest patients have v-tach just before they arrest. We're rarely there to see it but this time we had to treat it before shit went south. The treatment involved rapid defibrillation followed by IV and medication. It would either fix him or speed up the downhill process that he was already experiencing. It was only a matter of time before he went into cardiac arrest and I didn't want to see that. I was glad we got there when we did. Maddy got him on high concentration oxygen and got the intubation kit ready as I charged the defib. WEEEEEEEEEE, BEEP.

"CLEAR," I ordered, as everyone moved away. ZAPPPPPPP.

I discharged the machine and the old guy's frail body lurched a foot off the couch. He moaned after coming to rest. Billie, the engineman at 11 shouted, "Damn!"

The screen on the monitor took a second to refresh and afterwards showed no change. It was time for the second shock at the next higher power level. We'd do three times, if necessary. If he didn't improve we'd have to start CPR because v-tach doesn't allow enough blood to be pumped by the heart and you always shock first, and fast. WEEEEEEEE, BEEP. I zapped him a second time.

"DAMN " Billie said again. This time HE CONVERTED. The screen lit up and the old guy's heart was beating irregularly, but at least it was a rhythm. Now, it was time for an IV and a dose of Lidocaine to prevent him from going back into v-tach, then beat feet to the ER. The old guys eyes were wide open now and his skin color immediately improved. His breathing was back to normal and he spoke.

"My chest hurts," he muttered.

"I reckon it does, Pop, I reckon it does. You're gonna be OK. I'll get you an ice pack when we get outside," I said with relief. We got an IV in and gave him a dose of Lidocaine to suppress the chance of a recurrence of the deadly arrhythmia. After loading him into the unit, we sped to the ER without further incident. That was the first time I had ever shocked someone that was conscious. I had shocked many that didn't complain about their chest afterwards because they died. It was nice to hear one complain.

I saw Billie on another call, a couple shifts later. He said that that was the first time he'd seen a conscious v-tach patient "zapped" in his life. I said,

"Me too, Bill—me, too." Billie was one of my favorite enginemen. He was a big, rotund guy, that always seemed to be smiling, and seemed to like me. We would cut up on calls whenever we could, and always had a handshake and a hug for each other.

About a year after this "save," Billie was on another medical call. As they were taking a patient across the lawn to the ambulance, Billie collapsed. He had a massive heart attack and died on the way to the hospital, in the line of duty. It's hard to explain how this job allows you to get close people who you never really know, personally, away from the job. I'd never been to his house, never met his wife, kids, or grandkids (until the funeral), and never really knew him other than on the job, or seeing him at a union meeting on occasion. I lost a good friend and brother, though. I was hard to see Eleven roll up on a call without him after that because I missed him and still do. I'll never forget him, either.

Man Hater

I took the University of Maryland Fire Service Instructors Course shortly after I graduated from the academy. I figured that, if something happened to me, I'd have it to fall back on if I couldn't work in the field. This job has a tendency to cause bodily harm to you and I can't tell you how many times I'd get home from a shift and have a cut, scrape, or bruise, and have no idea how I got it. Hell, I'd never find it until I'd get in the shower, most of the time. Sometimes the injuries were more serious, like the cut on my arm in the "shitty" creek.

I had taken a short-course in mentoring and was qualified as a preceptor for newly hired paramedics or those who recently promoted from Cardiac Rescue Tech to NREMT-P. Maddy gave me the news that I would be detailed to Paramedic 12 for ten shifts, to precept my best friend, Brian. What the hell, it earned me an extra $400 when I was done.

I had met Brian at a party about twelve years earlier, when I first became a volly here in the county. My younger brother, Jess, was a volly at 13 and introduced me to him and Cuz at the same party. When I got hired by the county, Brian and I started hanging out together, mostly at "Happy Hour." We fished a lot together and he actually got me on as his mate when he ran a bay charter boat.

Brian was working at Paramedic 26 and had finally gotten his National Registry after being a CRT in the department for fifteen years. It was funny because he had been doing the job for about ten years longer than I had. It was going to be a fun, ten shifts, so I thought.

On our sixth shift together we got a call for an injured person. Waaaaaaaaaaahhhh……

"Medical Box 12-4, Paramedic 12 respond for an injured person from an assault, 1201 Earleigh Heights Road, cross street Jumpers Hole Road. county police en route." When the 911 operator judged the call to be non-urgent, they'd dispatch a medic unit only. We were a mile from this call. We arrived ahead of the police and were met outside of the residence by a male in his thirties.

"She's upstairs," he said, in a short blurt.

"Who is 'she' and what happened to her?" I asked, in a professional tone.

"She's my wife and we had an argument, OK?" he answered, angrily. He didn't appear injured and told us that *she* had initiated the call. I climbed the steps to the front porch and was greeted by a small child as I entered the front door. Brian followed with the trauma bag. I hated domestic calls like this where kids were involved.

I had separated from my wife two years earlier because we found ourselves arguing constantly. It wasn't healthy for the kids, who were twelve and three then. We agreed that being apart was better for them than subjecting them to that atmosphere, so I moved out. We remain friends to this day because, after all, she's the mother of my son. Some couples' entire relationships thrive on conflict and the kids, ultimately, suffer from it.

We were led to a second-floor bedroom by the small child and had directed the angry husband to wait outside for the police. When we entered the room we found the wife sitting on the edge of the bed, crying into a tissue.

"Hi," I said, as I sat on the bed next to her.

"I WANT THAT SON OF A BITCH LOCKED UP," she screamed.

"Now calm down, we're the paramedics. Are you injured?" I inquired, as I abruptly stood up. She didn't have any obvious signs of injury.

"OF COURSE I'M INJURED, THAT'S WHY I CALLED YOU," she scalded.

"OK, where are you injured, Ma'am," I said, in my professional tone. I could see that this was not going to be easy, but I kept my cool.

"RIGHT HERE," she scorned, as she pointed to the left side of her head. I attempted to inspect the site of the injury and she flinched away as soon as I touched her. I couldn't see an injury, or anything that resembled one, and thought her husband had probably just "bitch slapped" her, on the head.

"I WANT THAT SON OF A BITCH ARRESTED," she repeated. Now I'm getting pissed, but still keeping my professional tone.

"Ma'am, you'll have to take that up with the police when they arrive. Do you want to go to the hospital?" I asked.

"YES, YES," she shouted.

"OK, let's go," I ordered, as I helped her stand up.

"YOU DON'T CARE. YOU COULD CARE LESS ABOUT ME," she said, as she pulled her arm away from my outstretched hand.

A police officer entered the bedroom as we stood. I told him that the victim claimed to be assaulted but there were no obvious signs of an injury and she wanted to go to the hospital. He just gave me a funny look because he knew the routine better than I did.

"Ma'am, we're here to assist you in any way possible," I reinforced.

"BULLSHIT, YOU MEN ARE ALL ALIKE," she spat. Now I'm getting *highly* irritated and decide to take command of the situation.

"MA'AM, DO YOU WANT TO GO TO THE HOSPITAL OR NOT?" I said sternly. She staggered toward the bedroom door and I grasped her right upper arm firmly as she headed for the stairs. The last thing I wanted was this bitch falling down the steps and blaming me. She was obviously in her "anti-man" mode. Another cop was outside with the husband when we came out the front door.

Brian had gotten the stretcher out of the unit and rolled it to the bottom of the outside steps as we slowly started our descent. I still had her right arm and she held the aluminum railing with her left hand. Halfway down the steps, she does the old, "I'm going to faint" routine, and starts to fall forward. I knew it was an act because if she had truly fainted, her legs would have buckled and she would have melted down into a pile. I would have been able to pin her against the railing to keep her from going anywhere but, instead, she falls forward, almost like she was throwing herself down the steps. My reflex action was to spin around in front of her and slide my free hand under her left armpit, facing her. She was only a hundred pounds, wet, so I had her, until she lunged at me, trying to take me down the steps backwards with her. I tried to pull back, spin away, and let her dumb ass fall but she had my right hand pinned under her arm and I took all her weight against my extended right thumb. It hyper extended all the way back to my wrist.

"FUCK," I yelled, as I jerked my hand away from her and went to my knees in pain. Brian, who was stationed at the bottom of the steps, picked the bitch up like a sack of potatoes. He had her under his arm and carried her over to the unit, literally tossed her inside on the floor, then came to help me.

"Fuck man, I think it came out," I cried. My thumb had dislocated, then returned to its normal position after tearing all the connective tissue. It definitely HURT LIKE HELL. Brian called for an additional ambulance for the bitch, and wrapped my hand with an ice pack while we waited. I sat in the front seat next to him as he drove me to the ER, later.

After two months off and physical therapy twice a week, I was able to come back and finish Brian's last four shifts. I wanted to charge the psycho bitch with assault but couldn't prove that she purposely hurt me, which we all knew she did. I gave up after two more details. Being away from my shift, and partner wasn't worth the extra $400.

Back Home

Maddy and I had been working together for a couple of years. She had been having marital problems with her drunken husband and threw him out. She was an emotional train wreck and it was taking its toll on her.

Waaaaaaahhh…

"Medical Box 30-14, Engine 30, Paramedic 10 respond for a child in cardiac arrest, 2015 Outing Avenue, cross street 204th Street." This was every provider's nightmare and regardless of the age or circumstances, it was not going to be easy. Maddy was almost crying as I sped towards the call. If there was ever a time that we drove recklessly it was now but we always got there. I'm sure we generated complaints from the public at times that were squelched when the higher powers heard what the call was for.

Engine 30 arrived a minute ahead of us. They didn't advise us of the situation on the radio, so we figured they were busy. They were. We grabbed our equipment, ran into the house, and found 30's crew in a back bedroom. A male teenager was the only one present as we flew up the steps. The crew ran out to the living room with the child, who was limp and cyanotic (pale skin, blue lips, fingers and toes) and looked like he was about two years old. A firefighter was doing CPR as Maddy and I set up. I was going to intubate him and she was setting up for an IV. The EKG was a flat line and there were no signs of life.

The police, who routinely responded to all cardiac arrests, arrived and were interviewing the teen. He claimed to be the child's father and the mother's boyfriend. He stated that he heard a crash from the baby's room and, upon investigating, found the baby lying on the hardwood floor outside his crib. That was not likely because this baby had been dead for a while. I could tell that from the level of cyanosis and the fact that the story stunk, to me.

As I got ready to intubate the child, I noticed something. The child had four narrow bruises about three inches long across the right cheekbone.

"OFFICER, THIS CHILD HAS FACIAL TRAUMA THAT ISN'T CONSISTENT WITH A FALL FROM A CRIB," I barked, as I successfully planted the tube. The cop climbed the steps and I pointed to the obvious injury. He asked the teen to step outside. Maddy was just sitting there, on her knees, sobbing, and crying out loud.

"C'MON, WOMAN, I NEED YOU HERE," I commanded. Her hand was shaking as she made an attempt at the IV.

"TAKE THIS," I said to a firefighter, as he took over ventilations.

"GO," I barked at Maddy. She moved out of the way and, still kneeling, covered her face with her hands, sobbing, as I got the IV in. Maddy gathered herself enough to hand me medications from the bag when I asked for them, but that was all she could do. We never saw any heart activity during the entire call and I didn't think we would. The baby had been down too long before we arrived for us to help him and his head trauma was probably fatal, anyway.

We stopped CPR and ventilations long enough for me to run to the unit with the tiny, lifeless body. Some neighbors had gathered and they gasped and covered their faces as I ran by. The teen father was in handcuffs and was being led to the police car as we sped away.

The ER staff was ready when we arrived and they knew, too, that their efforts would probably be futile. The child was pronounced dead a short time later. The boyfriend, who was babysitting while the mother was in (high) school, admitted his guilt and told the police the real story. He had been feeding the baby, in his high chair, when the baby threw food at him. He tried to feed him again and the baby spit the food on him this time. The young father lost his temper and slapped the baby once, with an open hand, hard enough to knock over the high chair and the baby to the floor. He then panicked, picked the baby up, and took him to his crib then he cleaned up the mess and made up his story.

The outcome may have been the same, even if he had called us right away because who knows how long he waited to call—a senseless act. He would later receive a five-year sentence for involuntary manslaughter.

Maddy and I had the rest of the shift off, after the call. She would go home and take two more shifts off, to recover. I went to the bar, and was back the next shift.

Chapter 17
Heroes

I worked at Paramedic 10 for six years. It was my favorite assignment and my favorite crew. Maddy and I went through a lot in the three years that we worked together.

Waaaaaaahhh...

"Medical Box 10-06, Paramedic 10 respond to Maryland Medical Care, 2004 Mountain Road, cross street Magothy Beach Road for a cardiac."

Honestly, doctors' offices were a pain in the ass. Many times we were called to haul patients out to relieve the office of liability. When a patient would show up at their scheduled appointment with medical problems that required a higher level of medical tests or hospitalization, the staff would call us. Most of the time the problems these people had were chronic and not life-threatening, except this one.

Maddy and I arrived at the office, which was located in a shopping center a half mile from the station. We loaded our gear on the stretcher and rolled in. A staff nurse guided us to an exam room down a narrow hallway where we met a male in his forties. He was in atrial fibrillation, which is an irregularity that causes the atrium of the heart to beat out of sync. Although not as serious as ventricular fib, if it's not relieved, can lead to serious problems like a stroke or myocardial infarct (heart attack). This patient had the symptoms for two days, which made him a priority patient.

The staff nurse reported that his blood pressure was low and his heart rate was high. He, too, had "the look." He was pale and clammy and stated he felt weak. Maddy and I knew what we had to do but didn't want to do it in the doctor's office. We'd load him up first, then intervene. If shit went South, we'd be ready to roll because the procedure we were going to attempt had its risks.

We loaded the stretcher into the unit and prepped the patient. We were going to try to break the fib with medication first before administering a counter shock, which was a last resort and even more risky. The primary mission was to explain to the patient the procedure and what he was going to experience. Maddy had started an IV and I prepared the meds. The drug we were going to give was called Adenosine. Its success rate depended on your technique. If you didn't follow a certain sequence, or were a little slow in one of the steps, it probably wouldn't work. I calmed the patient and told him that he would feel like he was going to lose consciousness and assured him that we would not let anything happen to him. He took a deep breath and so did I. In a nutshell, Adenosine is a fast-acting, slow-lived drug that momentarily slows the heart to a near stop.

Most of the time this effect would allow the heart's electrical system to reset and get back into a regular rhythm. I had given it before and had good results, but the pucker factor was pretty high when you gave a patient a drug that was meant to stop his heart. Usually we're doing the opposite. The key to success was to push the drug then immediately follow it with a fast push of normal saline to move it quickly. If you were too slow with the initial push or slow with the flush, it wouldn't work. The IV line had a few med ports, which were rubber tipped entry points, to administer fluids and drugs. I stuck the Adenosine syringe, (which was only one cc) in the port closest to the IV site, and then I put a ten-cc syringe filled with saline in the next closest port. I'd warn the patient when I was ready to go and push the Adenosine, followed by the flusher. We closely monitored the screen on the EKG as we laid the patient flat.

"Ready?" I asked the patient. He nodded his head and took another deep breath. I closed the main IV line and pushed the small syringe, hard. I left it in the port and quickly pushed the saline. The patient eyes closed and he snored one time, deeply, as we watch his heart rate slow to a stop. My heart rate had doubled. We watched the flat line for about four seconds before the first contraction returned—then another—and another.

The man opened his eyes wide and said, "WOW." Gradually, his heart rate returned to normal and the fib was broken. Within a couple minutes the man's color returned and his respirations slowed. His heart rate was normal and he had a tear in his eye as he thanked us and gripped my hand. I felt good and fulfilled, I thought. It was times like this that made this job so satisfying and I wished I could feel it more often. It was like a good "buzz."

Two shifts later the EMS Battalion Chief McDonald, caught Maddy and I at the station. This was either a good thing or a bad thing. It was a good thing as he presented Maddy and I with two letters. The first was from our patient at the doctor's office. Surprisingly to us, he was a lieutenant with the Baltimore City Police Department, which he never mentioned. He also was a Maryland Army National Guard Medic. He praised our level of care, and our compassion. I was humbled. The second letter was a letter of commendation from Chief Timmons. "Attaboys" are a beautiful thing.

Meeting by Accident

I consider myself a good driver, on and off the job. My dad was a safety man at his job and always made everyone wear his or her seatbelts. He taught me how to drive by the example he set. Driving emergency vehicles is a challenge every time you roll out the door. Sooner or later bad luck would catch up to you, regardless.

Waaaaahhhhh...

"Medical Box 11-7, Paramedic 10, Paramedic 18, Ambulance 20, EMS 3 respond to assist Engine and Paramedic 11, on an auto accident, Fort Smallwood Road and Weldon Road. " We had heard the initial call go out and listened to the screaming on our station radio, as 11 arrived and the call evolved. We knew we were probably going to end up there and had our unit out the door as soon as Maddy grabbed the call printout from the printer. The vollies at 11 had their paramedic unit in service—otherwise we would have been on the original call. Paramedic 11 was the only volly unit in the county and had relocated from 28 about four years ago. Their personnel paled in comparison to the days when we ran it.

Volunteer Chief 11 had taken command and requested two additional medic units and one ambulance. This call had "circus" written all over it. He advised that there was a Priority One pediatric and adult patient as well as others less injured. It was just before five in the evening and we had thunderstorms roll through about forty-five minutes earlier. The travel portion of Fort Smallwood Road was dry but the center, left-turn lane, was still wet. I was driving, busting ass when I could, and that was the key to being a competent EVD (emergency vehicle driver). You had to know when to drive hard and when not to, lest you get bit in the ass.

Fort Smallwood Road was four lanes wide, with a center turn lane, where this accident had happened. There was a two-lane drawbridge over Stoney

Creek, just prior to the scene. I was "hauling the mail" across the bridge and as we approached the scene I noticed that both lanes of traffic were backed up. The police were making people do U-turns as they got close to the scene. The entire road was shut down.

I slowed from sixty to thirty as I exited the bridge and entered the center turn lane with the siren blaring and air horn blasting. They were gonna hear me coming, I thought. Traffic was backed up for a quarter of a mile as I eased past the stopped cars and saw the wreckage.

In a flash, a station wagon that was sitting in the line of traffic about halfway down the column bolted in front of us. I slammed on the brakes and tried to steer away from it, locking my arms on the steering wheel as we made contact.

BAAAAAAMMMMMMM

I saw the driver of the wagon fly across the front seat as we hit his door dead center. I still see it today like a bad flashback that won't go away. Debris flew onto the hood of the medic unit and the windshield shattered. My right arm was numb and my right shoulder throbbed with pain. Maddy had braced her arms on the dash and slumped down in the seat holding her neck. My first thought was to get to the driver that caused the crash. I had visions of a bloody corpse but I couldn't get my door opened.

Maddy was able to open her door and eased herself out of the vehicle. I climbed over the console and followed her as we both went to the passenger side of the wagon. The teenage driver was bleeding from his mouth and face as he lay on the bench seat of the wagon. Maddy supported his head and tried to control his airway. I sat on the ground near the rear of the car and called for help on the portable radio.

"PARAMEDIC 10 TO FIRE ALARM," I radioed.

"Paramedic 10."

"WE'VE BEEN INVOLVED IN AN ACCIDENT, A BLOCK FROM THE ORIGINAL CALL. DISPATCH A RESCUE BOX WITH AN ADDITIONAL BLS UNIT. WE ARE INJURED," I told them. There was silence. Apparently, the volly chief had covered my radio transmission and didn't even know we had crashed, even though we were within his sight.

"Paramedic 10, Chief 11 has command on the scene." They returned. FUCK! I repeated my call for help and this time the dispatcher heard me. Paramedic 18, who was dispatched with us on the original call for assistance, bypassed the original crash and came to us. Ambulance 20 did the same. The crew from 18 worked on the teenage driver as the crew from 20 helped us. More units were dispatched to the original call. In the service we called this a "Charlie Foxtrot," or military call words for CF (clusterfuck).

Paramedic 18 transported the teen to trauma with a serious facial injury. I hate to say this but, if the kid had his seat belt on, he would have been killed. The driver's door of his car had about eighteen inches of crush and that would have given him severe left side trauma. Instead, the impact threw him across the seat but, regardless, ALWAYS WEAR YOUR SEAT BELT. The chances of it saving you far outweigh the odds of it not.

The crew from Ambulance 20 had Maddy strapped to a board and took her away. Ambulance 30 had been dispatched and treated me likewise. All I could think about was the teen and whether I had done something wrong. I couldn't think straight. As I lay strapped to the board, waiting to get x-rayed at the ER, I went over the events leading to the crash, over and over. My head was spinning and I felt sick.

Twenty minutes seemed like hours before a doctor and a nurse came in and started removing straps and the board. They sat me up in a semi-reclined position. Chief McDonald came in and gave me a urinal bottle to piss in, which was SOP, he said. I complied and had nothing to fear. Fifteen minutes later he returned and advised me that the chain of custody was not in order and that I would have to wait for a lab tech to come to the ER. The kicker was, she was two hours away. I had to hold my bladder until then? I had just downed three cups of ice water, thinking I was done, and the CF continues. Make it stop, Mommy, please?

I asked McDonald about the crash investigation and he told me I was not at fault. The skid marks measured were twenty-two feet long, which put me at thirty-two miles per hour. The driver at fault had gotten impatient and had his front wheels turned sharply to the left, waiting for the car in front of him to move so he could make the illegal turn. That's why things happened so fast. The teen was going to be charged with "failure to yield right-of-way to an Emergency Vehicle" and "improper left turn." That didn't ease the pain a bit. I just hoped he would live.

I then inquired about the condition of the kid and people involved in the original call we were going to. He said neither patient was a Priority One, after all—we shouldn't have even been there. My bladder was the size of a basketball when I finally got to piss and the test results came back negative.

ther two months but this time I had my doctor keep me on pain
have to work light duty. I don't think I could've handled it.
...al therapy was painful and I still have occasional soreness in my
shoulder today. When I returned to work I put my transfer in for Paramedic
3, in the south. Paramedic 10 had just become a bad dream. The kid that caused
the accident was never charged.

Be Careful What You Wish For

In early '97 my transfer to Paramedic 3 was finally honored. I had to go
through administrative bullshit and file a grievance against the county to get it.
A medic from 18 had gotten in trouble and they needed to find a spot for him.
His transfer was filed after mine, which meant I had gotten bumped. It brought
back memories of the city. I needed out of 10 so I fought it and won. I wanted
that spot on "B" shift at 3 where I'd be working with a great medic named Brad
and, none other than, good old Ron. You may recall, Ron was the "brass hater"
that I worked with at the Heights, and then with Alan at 26.

Paramedic 10 was always known as the "night owl" unit. We were up after
midnight a lot, even when the busiest, 26, and 18 were lucky enough to catch
a slow night. It was a strange world after-hours. There was little or no traffic,
"barflys" and drunks, "weavin' and leavin'," and a quiet radio (except for us).
Paramedic 3 was slow at night and was generally known to be busiest while
the many doctors' offices and health care facilities surrounding the city of
Annapolis were open. Trust me, there were a ton of them, and I welcomed the
thought of finally working on a unit where I could, at least, go home in the
morning and not have to go to bed.

Station 3 was a huge, older volunteer station. There weren't any active
volunteer members that rode anymore but there were still administrative
vollies. They were very good to us. The station was a three-story brick building
that had four bays that faced Riva Road. If you drove around the to back of
the building, there were three more bays on a lower level that faced the local
Post Office. It housed Engine 3, Engine 3-2 (the volly engine that just collected
dust), Tanker 3, Brush 3 (a mini-pumper), Utility 3 (a Ford pickup), Boat 3 (a
seventeen-foot Boston Whaler, on a trailer) and Paramedic 3. The building
was full.

Call volume in the county was ever-increasing. Every year the number of
medical calls would increase by at least ten percent. The city of Annapolis Fire

Department had three stations, each with medic units. Station 39 was located near the U.S. Naval Academy and first due into the historic downtown district. Station 35 was located on the west side of town and very near the county line. Station 36 was located in the Eastport section of town and about halfway between the other two. For the longest time Annapolis only had two medic units. When an increase in development and booming business interests moved in, Paramedic 36 was placed in service. Up until then, Paramedic 3 was like a supplemental unit for the city, running almost as many calls there as they did in the county. We always had a great working relationship with the guys from the city. Hell, Engine 3 was slow most of the time, so we ran more calls with the city guys than we did our own.

The working relationship between the suppression people and the medics at 3, was strange. Being at a slow station made them lazy, I guessed. The medic unit ran a lot during the day and slowed down at night. Basically, the engine and tanker sat a lot, always. It didn't have the same feel as it did at 10. It didn't feel like family. Brad and I had worked at 10 together for a year or so before he split for Three. We made it fun to work together.

We'd stay on the street just to stay away from the station. The place was depressing. We'd cruise the mall and the Harbor Center, then ride around our first due area checking out the local beaches. We spent a lot of time on the street, which meant we spent a lot of time together. Brad was smart and had a great sense of humor, like me. We were two peas in a pod and worked well together. For the first time in my career I could actually say that I had fun at work. I dreaded working with Ron but after getting his ass busted for his attitude at the Heights and an incident at 26, he was a little more low key than he had been in the past. He was still irritating at times.

Within three months of my arrival at 3, things changed. For some unknown reason we were getting busier at night. Everyone was, actually. Our first due area was huge and sometimes an advanced life support call after midnight would mean a two-hour turn-around time. Our area stretched from the city (Annapolis), some twelve miles to the neighboring county and six miles east and south to the peninsula and the Bay. The closest hospital was located downtown in Annapolis and could be, at times, a thirty minute drive for us, depending where the call was located.

Brad and I would run our calls and travel to the other stations to cook or eat our meals (if we didn't eat on the street). We ran with them more than our home station, too. Station 2 was located near the beach and was our second home. Station 40, next to the mall, was the company we ran with the most. They were our families. Three was just a miserable place to be. The captain was unhappy about his assignment and didn't like the guys assigned to him, and the guys were unhappy because they didn't like the captain—and none of them liked us (yes, *more* haters). Maybe it was because we'd forget to reset the radio to silent mode when we got a call in the middle of the night and they'd have to get up to do it. Well, sometimes we forgot, just to piss them off. After all, we were working and they were sleeping.

Exemplary Performance?

One shift, Brad, and Ron were off and I worked with JC, from "A" shift. He was senior to me and had been in the department for quite some time. He was cool to work with and he was a fisherman, like me. We heard Engine 5 dispatched to set up a landing site (LZ-landing zone) for a med-evac from Squad 7 and Paramedic 5. They had run a crash on Chesterfield Road at the "End-of-the-World" hill. It was a straight, narrow, two-lane road that suddenly plummets down a mile and a half-long, windy-ass hill, through a forest leading down to the South River—hence the name.

Years ago, Mel and I used to get liquored up and purposely launch his sister's '69 Impala off the thing. It was a "tank" and would only go airborne for about twenty feet, but it was funny as shit (it caught fire and burned up one day because the catalytic converter and muffler had been smashed against the floorboard and, one day, ignited the carpet). Wonder how that happened. Paramedic 5 was calling help.

Waaaaaaahhhh…

"Rescue Box 7-31, Paramedic 3 respond, Priority 1, to assist Squad 7 and Paramedic 5 on an auto accident with entrapment, Chesterfield Road, cross street Saint Stephens Church Road."

JC and I rolled out the door. It sounded like a pretty bad crash from the radio transmissions we heard while en route. The volly chief from 7 was in command, which meant things were going to be hectic when we got there. Are you noticing a pattern here? That's all I'm going to say about that. We had gotten our assignment prior to arriving and when we arrived, went to work. The medics from 5 were split up, meaning they had two priority patients. All of our medic units carried enough equipment and supplies that we could each work independently, if necessary. A sixteen-year-old male had launched his Honda Prelude off "the Hill." Who can say whether he did it purposely or was just going too fast in the wrong place? At any rate, the Honda flew over a hundred feet before it hit, spun sideways, and rolled another hundred. The driver was out of the car and being attended to by the crew from Ambulance 7. The driver's fourteen-year-old girlfriend was seated in the front seat and was trapped so JC went to the car. Her twelve-year-old brother was riding in the back seat and was ejected through the back window during one of the rolls. I grabbed a trauma bag and went to him. It wasn't pretty.

The medic from 5 that was working on the victim gave me a quick rundown. He was fairly new to the department and had his hands full working alone. He tried to be cool as he spat out his observations. The young victim was barely breathing and the medic from 5 was bagging him. I saw blood coming from the boy's ears and noticed that his right pupil was "blown" (fully dilated and not reactive to light). This kid had a serious skull fracture, a brain injury and, more than likely, a spinal cord injury judging from his lack of neuro function. We had to move fast and the other injuries to his extremities were closed fractures and didn't warrant our attention right now. With a cervical collar already in place (it's the first thing we do), we strapped him to a backboard and trucked up the hill toward Paramedic 3, which someone had moved closer to us.

I could hear Trooper 8 circling the LZ, which was located at the top of the hill in a field. Once in the unit, I got an IV started on the kid and scribbled vital signs and observations on a note pad. As we headed for the LZ, I radioed Johns Hopkins Pediatric Trauma Center and gave them the patient info. There wasn't much else we could do but get this kid there, ASAP. We stopped in the field, a safe distance from the chopper. The idling bird was waiting to fly as the flight medic opened the back doors of our unit. This was one of the few times that he would look at us and say, "C'mon, let's go," without even climbing on board. He knew we had to go. We transferred *our* board to the special helicopter board and four of us carried the fragile load to the waiting chopper, as the medic from 5 continued bagging. He would fly with them today, since he was the initial primary provider. This kid was his. The flight medic slid the cabin door shut and secured it. I tapped him on the shoulder and gave him a thumbs up before trotting to a safe spot during lift-off. Trooper 2 was on the way for the driver and his girlfriend. They would take both of them to Shock Trauma but their injuries weren't as serious as the youngster's.

After the second helicopter took off, JC and I gathered our equipment and headed for home. We had a mess to clean up and reports to write. I got a phone call not long after we returned. It was the medic from 5 calling to let me know that as soon as Trooper 8's wheels left the grassy field, the kid coded. Hopkins worked on him for a while before pronouncing him dead. I was disappointed, but not shocked.

We have people who are critically injured all the time. We do what we can and send them off. Rarely are the outcomes good. We just do our job the best we can and pray for the best. The "Higher Power" is always in control. About two months later, JC told me that we were getting a "unit citation" and decorated for "exemplary performance."

"Why?" I asked.

"The kid died. Gimme an award for saving someone, huh?" I added. I didn't understand and was required to accept the award. It didn't make sense to me and I would soon learn that the awards committee of the department was a joke, anyway. Every year people would get awards for stupid shit while a lot of deserving people got denied. It was very political and if someone on the committee didn't like you, you didn't get squat. It would be my first, and last award.

I received campaign ribbons for Hurricanes Floyd, Isabel, and the "Blizzard of 2003," but that was because I showed up for work and finished the shifts without getting killed or injured.

Firefighting

One thing about working in the south end of the county was, the stations were farther apart which meant if you had a fire, your help took a little longer to get there. It made for exciting times. I did a lot more firefighting at 3 than anywhere else. Of course by now, our staffing levels were down and medics were called on to supplement the firefighting force more often. The implementation of a RIT (Rapid Intervention Team) by the NFPA had all of our people in a tiff.

A RIT consisted of two firefighters in full gear with masks and a charged hose line at the front door of the fire building. If you were the first to arrive, you could not make an attack on a fire until the RIT was in place. If you had a confirmed rescue (someone hanging out of a window, screaming, with fire licking their ass), that was the only exception.

Our engines were staffed with an average of three people. A couple stations were lucky and had four or had vollies and could load up. Some only had two on an engine, which was insane. What's even more insane? The county has sent engines out the door with driver only for years. I guess their mentality is it looks better having something sitting in front of the fire, doing nothing, as opposed to showing up a few minutes later. The union has been trying to stop that practice ever since I can remember. OK, let's do some math.

*Engine 3 is first due on a dwelling fire.

*They have three heads—a driver, an officer, and a firefighter.

*They get to the scene and have a room and contents, like a bedroom or kitchen, off.

*They can't go in and put the fire out until Engine 40 or Engine 2 gets there and drags a second line to the front door. (Remember that the pump operator can't leave the engine.) Sometimes that would take five minutes or more. If Engine 3 were lucky, Paramedic 3 wasn't at a nursing home or doctor's office and would be right there with them from the git-go. See where I'm going with this? The bottom line was, we were understaffed. I'm not sure *waiting* for a RIT was safer than going in and knocking down the fire before it intensified. It should be a judgement call by the officer but not a requirement. After all, they did it for over 200 years and now, your officer can't make a decision. I'll stick with the "meat wagon," thank you.

Hurricane Floyd

The third major hurricane of the 1999 Atlantic season was named Floyd. The department prepared as it churned up the East Coast. It was scheduled to hit on *our* shift and had already dumped, some sixteen inches of rain on North Carolina. I have worked during several of them over the years and to me, it was just a wet and windy pain in the ass. People here in the Mid-Atlantic call them hurricanes, but they are rarely more than a tropical storm by the time they reach us in Maryland. We've had true hurricanes in the past but they were rare. The most famous one here was in 1933 and actually cut what is now known as, the Ocean City Inlet.

I was excited about anything that kept me out of a doctor's office and Brian and I were ready. We had our rain gear on, early, and made sure the fuel tanks on the unit were full. The power at the station went out early and the engine was running downed wires all morning. We ran a crash in the morning and drove the old lady involved to Shock Trauma. There would be no helicopters today. It was Sunday and in the early afternoon we ran a dwelling fire where the resident just had to watch football. His power was out and he didn't have a generator so he plugged his little portable TV into the cigarette lighter of his car, in the garage. He left the set unattended for a few minutes and when he returned, the car was on fire. Apparently something got hot or shorted out and in an attempt to extinguish the blaze himself, received some serious burns. It was then that he called 911. When we arrived, the garage and half the house were lit.

Please learn from this. CALL 911 IMMEDIATELY AND GET OUT. A lot of people think they can fight the fire themselves and actually lose precious minutes, and most of their belongings. A matter of ten minutes can make a difference. If the fire is small and you have a hose or extinguisher handy, try to put it out, but ONLY after you have called 911. This man's actions earned him a trip to the Burn Center, but he survived. After returning from our second trip to Baltimore, we ran a service call to one of the local nursing homes. They had lost power, had no generator, and were worried that their patients that had to be on oxygen full time, would run out. I made a call to the duty officer to arrange to have a few large bottles of oxygen delivered to them. It was then— I heard a familiar voice on the radio.

"ENGINE 23 TO FIRE ALARM, WE'VE JUST BEEN INVOLVED IN AN ACCIDENT, RITCHIE HIGHWAY AND ARNOLD ROAD. CHECKING PERSONNEL FOR INJURIES. NO OTHER VEHICLES INVOLVED."

IT WAS KEVIN! He had transferred to the haz-mat unit and was the lieutenant at 23. We were the closest unit to them.

"Paramedic 3 to Fire Alarm, clearing this call, en route to assist 23," I rang out. It was raining like hell. Twenty-three was responding to a call when a hundred-foot-tall oak tree fell across Ritchie Highway, right in front of them. The driver did a great job missing the tree but skidded into the median strip. The heavy engine was no match for the soft ground and flipped onto its side in the grass. By the grace of the Gods, not one of the guys were hurt. Imagine the sickening feeling we had when we rolled up and saw that.

"KEVIN, YOU ALL RIGHT?" I shouted, as I walked towards him, briskly. He just shook his head. His eyes were the size of saucers. I patted him on the back as we embraced.

"Goddam, Boy, you scared the shit out of me," I scorned.

"YOU? HOW DO YOU THINK I FELT?," he spouted. We laughed and, one-by-one, Brian and I embraced our brothers. No matter what happened for the rest of the shift, this was a good day. Brian and I would go to Trauma one more time before it was all over. A man just *had to* get on his roof and clear the rain gutters of debris. A gust of wind knocked him off the roof. He fell about twelve feet, landing in the grass, a foot from the basement stairwell. I got home at eight the next morning and slept for fourteen hours.

My Miracle Kid

If I ever experienced a miracle, it was now. It was a quiet Sunday morning in May, so let's get to it.

Waaaaaaaaahhhh...

"Medical Box 40-24, Engine and Ambulance 40, Paramedic 3, respond for an auto accident at Generals Highway and Bestgate Road, in front of the Annapolis Mall."

Any of the many intersections around the massive mall were dangerous. They were the scene of a hundred, or so, accidents a year. Most of them were minor because of the congestion and people's inability to get any speed up. This morning was different as Forty arrived we heard this on our radio.

"ENGINE 40 TO FIRE ALARM, MSP HELICOPTER FOR AN EIGHT-YEAR-OLD

WITH SEVERE MULTI-SYSTEMS TRAUMA—PARAMEDIC 3 EXPEDITE" One thing about this job, that I learned a long time ago, was never taking things for granted. At any time, on any day or night, you might be subject to the most horrible call you could ever imagine. There was no traffic on this morning and my foot was nailed to the floor. The intersections on Riva Road were wide and I blew through each one with total disregard, red light or not. Brian was blasting the air horn as we rocketed toward the scene.

As we arrived, we saw a silver Volvo station wagon that had been struck broadside by a Chevy Suburban, on the passenger side. A woman was standing near, as was a teenage boy. A well-dressed man stood next to the rear passenger door of the wagon, which was partially opened. Brian grabbed the airway kit and I grabbed the trauma bag and oxygen.

We ran toward the car. The lieutenant from 40 rambled something about a trauma doctor and said the family was on their way to church. They didn't see the oncoming truck. I looked past him and saw a little boy lying across the rear seat. He had a massive facial injury, his right eye socket was fractured, and the eye was unstable. The right side of his face, including his mouth, was severely mutilated. His only movements were during his labored gasps for air. The well-dressed man spoke.

"I'm Doctor (whatever) from Trauma," he said calmly.

"MOVE," I ordered, as Brian and I bent the crushed door open as wide as possible. He stepped away.

"He needs to be intubated. Do you have a tube?" the doctor inquired.

"HE NEEDS A COLLAR AND AN AIRWAY FIRST. WHAT ARE WE DOING HERE?" I said sharply. Nothing, that I could see, but standing around waiting for me. *Get, the fuck, out of my way—I've got shit to do,* I thought to myself. I bit my tongue.

"I'll ride with him in the helicopter," he said.

"He's going to the closest ER, five minutes down the street. This kid needs an airway. MIKE, CANCEL THE TROOPER, WE'RE GOING TO ANNE ARUNDEL," I demanded, shouting at the lieutenant. I gently and quickly slid a collar on the child's neck as Brian handed me a child-sized bag mask. I began to move air into his lungs. A quick look revealed no other obvious injuries except the right side of the child's face, which looked hideous.

Brian readied the appropriate sized tube. It would be a "blind digital" attempt (you use your fingers to open the airway, instead of using a metal blade to visualize the airway, then you slide the tube over the fingers, blindly). It was difficult to do in training, let alone now. The doctor made the first attempt.

"I don't think it's in," he stated, as he slowly removed it and stepped away.

"OK, LET'S ROLL BOYS," I commanded. "WE'RE OUTTA HERE." I stopped bagging just long enough to grasp the child under his arms. Brian supported his head and we slid the child onto the waiting board and stretcher and rolled to the unit.

"You coming?" I asked the doctor. He shook his head and I slammed the door closed.

"GET US THERE, ERIC," I shouted through the sliding cab window. The firefighter from 40 knew we had little time. He gassed on it. I was happy that it was Eric because he was a great guy to work with and knew how to get us there fast without tossing us around, like BB's in a shoebox. I went back to bagging.

Although the injury to the child's face looked bad, there was very little external bleeding. I knew he had blood entering his airway and occasionally used the suction unit to try to keep it clear. I spoke to him softly but firmly.

"Hang in there, little buddy. We're taking care of you," I said. It was a habit all good medics had, to talk to your patient, even if they're unconscious. There's no way to know if they can hear you, but it can't hurt. Some people that recover actually say they remember hearing a voice talking to them. It helped *me* deal with the moment, too.

Brian had placed the EKG pads and was ready to try another intubation. The child's vital signs were normal and so was his EKG. That was surprisingly good news and I hoped his brain was OK. I stopped bagging as Brian tried the tube. Once again, we weren't sure it was in. I was moving air well with the bag so we were content with bagging for a couple more minutes. I continued encouraging the little guy to be tough. My emotions were catching up with me. Eric backed us into the ER bay as the awaiting staff opened the rear doors. We swept the child into the trauma room like lightning. I helped the nurses remove his shoes and clothing and that's when it hit me.

My son Michael was nine and this kid was eight. That was close—too close. Everything I removed from him reminded me of Michael—his little digital watch, his woven leather belt, his shoes with the Velcro straps, his dress slacks, everything.

I remembered the times that Michael would fall asleep in the car or on the couch and I'd carry him to his room. I'd get him out of his clothes and into his pajamas without waking him. I wondered if *this* little guy was going to wake up. I so wished he would. I crumbled then I bailed.

"I gotta go," I choked, as I briskly turned and bolted from the room. A nurse followed me and grabbed my shoulder.

"Are you alright?" she asked.

"No. I'm not," I admitted. She put her arm around me and walked me outside.

"I just saw my son lying there," I sobbed. She hugged me tighter.

"It's not, Mark. It's not him," she assured. "Just stay out here and relax for a minute. You guys did a great job," she added. I felt better, but couldn't get the images out of my head. I started working on getting our equipment back in service but, after a few minutes, found myself trying to do six things at once. I couldn't focus on any *one* thing. I knew I was through for the shift. Brian knew it, too. I guess it was easier for him to deal with because he didn't have kids.

I sent Brian into the room every five minutes, to keep me up on the kid's status. The ER doctor had gotten a tube in, the nurses had started an IV, and they had given him Mannitol, which decreases any swelling there might be in the brain. It sounded like he was stabilizing. I sobbed again.

Paramedic 9 arrived with a patient and the ER staff immediately informed them of the situation and the need for a medic unit to transfer the child to Baltimore. Dan, the crew chief on 9, called Communications and informed them that they would be transferring the child to Hopkins Pediatric Trauma. There was no time to go through administrative channels and I prayed that the child would make the trip. Johns Hopkins is the best children's hospital in the world, bar none.

"If he makes it there, he'll be OK," I assured myself. I prayed for him and I was afraid for his life. I got back to the station and gathered my gear. My relief person was on the way but I was free to go when I was ready. The first thing I did, before I left the parking lot at 3, was to call Michael. When I heard his voice, I almost lost it. I asked him if he was OK.

"Yeah, why Daddy?" he inquired.

"Just wondering, buddy," I said, with a choke.

"How's things with you?" he asked.

"I'm OK. I just needed to hear your voice, that's all," I said softly.

"Oh, OK," he said. "Well, here I am," he said with a chuckle. He had no idea. I told him I loved him and hung up. I sat in the parking lot and cried for five minutes before I could leave. He must have thought I was weird or something. I'd tell him about the call the next time I saw him. I'd give him a "bear hug" until he complained, and he'd comfort me just by being alive. I couldn't imagine losing him. I know it would kill me.

The following shift, I checked the time sequence for the call. We received the call and were on the scene in five and a half minutes. We were *at* the scene for seven minutes (seemed longer, didn't it?) and were at the hospital in five minutes. It was a total of seventeen and a half minutes from the time we got the call until we arrived at the hospital. I felt like a super hero because that was an incredible feat and amazing times.

We blew the "Golden Hour" away. Trauma experts call the first hour after a severe injury, the most critical. During this hour, lives are in the balance, and saved or lost, depending of course, on their severity, and the echelon of care available. The most amazing thing was, the little guy was getting better by the day. I checked on him every shift for a month. He didn't lose his eye. He had reconstructive surgery to his face and had a lot of work to do relearning words and speech due to his brain injury, but I knew he was a tough guy, like me, and would be OK.

The story of his recovery hit the front page of the local paper a few weeks later. "A Miracle," the caption read. Indeed it was. His mother had sent us a wonderful letter, praising God and us. We received a letter of commendation from the chief of the department. The lieutenant from Engine 40 had recommended Brian and I for a unit citation and exemplary performance award. It was denied for the following reason—"They were just doing their job." The trauma doctor, at the scene, was given a citizen's exemplary performance award—congratulations. What a joke.

The Annapolis Firefighter's Emerald Society held a fundraiser for the child and his family at "Heroes," our favorite watering hole. It would help them with their monumental medical bills. I tried to bring myself to go to the event and see him, but I couldn't. I was scared to death. I was afraid I'd see him and make a blubbering fool of myself. I realized I was still recovering, too. I hope he gets to read this someday. I know he'd understand and, one day, I'll see him.

September 11, 2001: The Worst Shift of My Career

It started out like any normal shift. We had an ORI (Operational Readiness Inspection) scheduled for the next week so we had to make sure our stuff was right. We had our unit's reputation to uphold and each shift was assigned a particular part of the medic unit to clean and stock. Our shift's job was the exterior. We had to wash, wax, and polish the paint, chrome, and aluminum. Our new unit was big so I had to get on a twelve-foot stepladder to wax the bugs off of the front of the box, above the cab.

That's when the news came. The tanker driver came out and told me I had to see this report on TV. A commercial jetliner had crashed into the World Trade Center in Manhattan. I just thought it was an accident and recalled the plane that hit the Empire State Building back in the 1940s or 1950s. I wanted to get the wax off that I had already applied, so I continued my task for a few minutes longer. When I finally got down off the ladder and walked into the TV room, the second plane was about to hit. *This was no accident, I* immediately thought.

The room was silent as the minutes ticked by. No one spoke a word. We just sat there watching as word came in of the Pentagon attack, then the peril of Flight 93 in Pennsylvania. What was happening to our world? I wondered. Headquarters had ordered all stations to lock down. This was surreal. We hung our heads when the first tower fell. Every one of us knew what had just happened because we knew our brothers were in there. I tried to picture them in my mind, climbing flight after flight of steps. It was going to take over an hour for the first ones to reach the eighty-fourth floor. With all their gear and any equipment they carried with them, they'd go three or four stories and have a "blow," then three or four more, and stop again—for over an hour. Then came the task of fighting the fire and making rescues. I thought about my days at the academy, and the bowling alley fire, when climbing to the top of the ladder truck winded me. That was only nine or ten stories and it made my chest hurt. It was hurting for a different reason today.

When the second tower fell, all of our hopes fell with it. We knew the civilian body count would be high but had no idea that the FDNY had lost most of an entire shift and all of their equipment. I was sick to my stomach and realized that I had never felt hatred towards anyone, until that day. Now I know what it feels like to hate someone. I hate the people who committed this act of cowardice. I will NEVER forgive them and I hope that they die as brutally as did every innocent soul that day. Anyone that disagrees with me or thinks that these barbarians deserve "rights" can kiss my ass. It's "kill or be killed" with these people and I say, fight for our fallen brothers and our freedom. No half-assed, fanatical religious group that threatens me, my family, friends, countrymen, and most importantly, my freedom, should be allowed to live. They live like rats in the mountains of Afghanistan. They need to be exterminated like the rodents they are.

My dad is a veteran of the Korean War and a Life Member of the American Legion. My mom was in the Women's Army Corp. My grandfather and half-a-dozen of my uncles are veterans. They, and thousands of our ancestors, fought for the freedom and the rights we have today. I'll be damned if I'll allow some punk-assed, camel jockey, named Usama Bin Laden, threaten to take it away. For the sake of all those who gave their lives to protect it, so shall we. Anyone that disagrees with this is not a true American and can move out of MY country. Any politician that disagrees should be impeached and exiled. "GOD BLESS AMERICA." "LET US NEVER FORGET." Now, you wanna know how I really feel?

Brian and I ran nonstop the entire shift. We ran everything from panic and anxiety attacks, to stress-related chest pains, along with all the regular stuff. We finally got to bed around three AM after twenty hours in hell, and it wasn't over. At 5:45 we got a call for a self-inflicted gunshot wound. I'm not giving the details on this one because it hurts to recall it. The call was at the exclusive home of a government defense contractor that had lost most of his employees at his office at the Pentagon. He was distraught and felt guilty that he wasn't there with them. He's with them now. God bless them all.

Brian and I were silent as we cleared the call and headed for the station. We were mentally and physically spent. The worst shift of our career was finally over.

Chapter 18
The Beginning of the End

A lot of things were transpiring in my life—both of them. I wasn't happy at work and it was taking its toll on me at home. Emergency Medical Services, nationwide, was changing and it was a change I couldn't deal with. I wasn't alone because morale in the department was at an all-time low. The most critical phrase that people would use in describing the fire department administration was, "While the ship is sinking, they're rearranging the deck furniture." I heard people use that one from day one and sadly, it was true.

I was changing, too. I had over seventeen years of service with the county when I started planning my escape. I was facing the facts and, when all was said and done, I had gotten to the point where I didn't want to do the job anymore. I was burning out. After twenty-plus years, the fire inside me was dying. We went nine years, in the late 1980s and early 1990s without a cost-of-living raise. Sure, we got other concessions but nothing that showed up in the paycheck every week. It was catching up with the administration and there was no simple solution. Five- and ten-year veterans of the department were quitting and starting over with other departments that paid better and had different work schedules. We had a lower starting salary and pay scale than all the other departments in the Baltimore-Washington, D.C. region.

Medics, myself included, were fed up with the "new and improved," "kinder, gentler" fire department that was evolving. Someone came up with a thing called "Quality Assurance" and "Customer Service." This isn't a fucking WalMart, it's a fire department. It was killing what little morale was left. In a nutshell, it meant that roving supervisors would be assigned to randomly run from call to call and evaluate your level of care and, if they thought it was necessary, give you a counseling notice or at the least, a critique. Most of the time it was only to justify their position. Unfortunately, the people that they put in these positions were the incompetents that they had pulled off the street because they were a liability.

In the course of my career I received twenty-three letters of commendation. I was decorated by the county, got awards from the city of Baltimore, MIEMSS, the United Way, the AFL-CIO and IAFF, The Baltimore Regional Burn Center, and every volly company I was ever a member of. At one time, I was the youngest of only three volunteer EMS lieutenants officially recognized by the county. I was a mentor, a preceptor, and still am a qualified Fire Service Instructor with the University of Maryland. I have my CDL with every endorsement possible including motorcycle. I'm a U.S. Coast Guard Licensed Captain and never got less than a Level 1 (the highest) Performance Evaluation every year, until the last year of my career. The last thing I needed was some incompetent fuck following me around telling me how to do my job, and a job that I'd done well for over twenty years. Did I ever make a mistake in the field? Everyone does sooner or later, especially if you've been running calls for twenty hours straight. If you're in the service and haven't yet, *you will*, trust me on that one. Did I ever generate any complaints? You have to, and every good medic will. If you don't, people will walk all over you, and half of our calls involved a drunk or an idiot, anyway.

If your six-year-old gets a fever, give him some Tylenol and take him to the fucking doctor. Don't call 911 at two in the morning (because you just got home from the bar) for a free taxi ride to the ER. If you cut your finger making dinner and need stitches, wrap a fucking paper towel on it and go to the ER. Don't call 911 for a ride because you don't want to sit in the waiting room with a bunch of sick "illegals" or think you'll get faster service if you call me. I'll "rat" your ass out with the triage nurse and you'll end up in the waiting room anyway. Here are some more words of advice. Don't try to fake being unconscious or fake a seizure. We have ways of figuring you out and some of them involve painful stimuli. Save yourself the pain and suffering and talk to me. I'm smarter than you think and there's a good chance I'm smarter than you are.

If you're a medical professional remember this, SO AM I. Just because you think I ride around in a truck with lights and a siren, and give people rides to the hospital doesn't mean we can't talk about bruits, an abdominal aortic aneurysm, or placenta previa. I was in the crushed, overturned vehicle, with gasoline leaking everywhere, starting an IV, fifteen minutes before I delivered the patient to your well-lit, well-stocked, sterile place of employment.

People have the ability to test your nerves in this business and they will every chance they get. These were just a few of the things that might get us off on the wrong foot. My point is, if you play me for a fool, insult my intelligence, abuse the 911 system, clog up an ER with shit calls that your doctor can handle, or tell me you've only had one beer when I know you've been drinking all day, we're gonna have a problem. Of course the department policy now is "the customer is always right." If you call and make up some bullshit story about how I treated you badly or said something that hurt your feelings, they'll believe you, even if you're a lowlife piece of shit. It happened to more than one of us and that was another department morale buster—the "guilty until proven innocent" mentality, which was total bullshit. Whatever happened to the idea of having a little faith and trust in your "quality" people, or does the quality of your recent, newly-hired employees really suck that bad?

With the call volume increasing and no additional units being placed in service, along with all the other bullshit, every unit was busy and overtime was plentiful. The trouble was, no one wanted to work. Hell, no one wanted to work their regular shift, let alone overtime. Annual leave was being cancelled left and right, and if your relief called in sick and no one would want to work, you were "held over." Holdover had been around for quite a while but was totally out of control by now. Someone from EMS got held over almost every day, and weekends were the worst. This was the final blow that finished me off. There was a rotational calendar and everyone was assigned a number. If your number was up for the next day and a slot (could be anywhere in the county) couldn't be filled, you were held over. If it came up on a Friday, Saturday, or Sunday you were screwed. Got plans for your first day off? Tough shit. Got a doctor's appointment? It sucks to be you. Got to pick your kid up from daycare because your wife is working late? Sorry about your luck. Have a part-time business on your days off? Too bad. Does your kid have a soccer game? Sorry, you missed it. Do you know what the killer was? If you were up all night running calls and got zero hours of sleep, then got held over, it was "Oh, well." That's where I drew the line and it happened to me, once. I vowed, never to let it happen again.

I had been up all night at 3. I slept in a recliner for an hour and a half because I was too tired to climb the steps to the bunkroom. My holdover number was on for the next day and someone called in sick. They couldn't fill the spot so I was held over for another twenty-four hours. Where's the "Quality Assurance" here? Myth: "Oh, 9 is slow, you'll be able to get some sleep there." Truth: Bullshit. You can not sleep at *ANY* firehouse during the morning hours because of vacuum cleaners, phones ringing, dumb asses that "forget" you're in there sleeping, intercoms, and, oh yeah, let's not forget calls.

I arrived at 9 and went directly to the bunkroom, demanding not to be disturbed as I stumbled through the kitchen. Twenty minutes after I lay down, we got a call for a child that fell through a storm door and was injured. I was pissed and my head was spinning like a top. I was trying to mentally prepare for the worst scenario, as I would on any call, but I couldn't. I pictured this kid, sliced from asshole to appetite, tried to plan an attack, and I couldn't do it. My brain was locked up. I was so fatigued I couldn't think.

Fortunately, the child's injury was minor. I called the EMS duty officer from the hospital and told him that I was finished.

"You can fire me if you want, and I'll see you in court, but I'm gonna end up killing someone, if not myself. This unit is out of service, as of right now," I warned. I probably shouldn't have driven home, I was that tired. They didn't fire me. It was insane for me to be there because I was a lawsuit looking for a place to happen. It didn't make any sense and the shit really hit the fan when two of our medics from 17 spilled the beans to a reporter from the local paper. The front page headline the next day read, "Paramedic Fatigue.... Are You Really Safe?" The uncertainty of not knowing whether I could go home at the end of an ass-kicking, twenty-four-hour shift made me want to quit. It was crazy, and opposite of the whole "QA" and "customer service" bullshit they had us doing—BUT IT WAS LEGAL. The law stated that they could force me to work, regardless of my physical and mental status.

I put my transfer in for Paramedic 1 the following shift. It was the slowest medic unit in the county (relatively speaking). One's first due area bordered 3's, to the South. I had to stop the madness. I finally faced the fact that I was burned out, and it hurt.

I spent a total of nineteen months in the Baltimore City fire department. I was hired by Anne Arundel County with no interruption of employment. The state allowed a transfer of service credit from one department to another within the state, with that stipulation. Therefore, I should "get out of jail" nineteen months early, plus, any accrued sick leave I had would be credited towards my retirement date as well. That was the rumor, anyway.

Baltimore City advised that I was a probationary employee with them for the first year and that was not really service time because I didn't contribute to their pension fund. In other words, service does not mean service, it means

. I'm glad we got that cleared up. I ended up getting seven months of service credit transferred and it was more bullshit, but not worth the headache fighting it. I was tired of all the politics that had already cost me enough in wage concessions over the years. I just want to ride off into the sunset. If I used the word bullshit a lot, I'm sorry, that's what it amounted to.

Many people in the department thought that sick leave was "special vacation" leave and burned it as soon as they accumulated it. That was a bad move, especially if you did anything sports-related on your days off, or had a small business involving physical labor (remember, I burned all the sick leave I had accumulated for four years when I blew my knee up playing softball). I had six months of sick leave saved up. I was rarely ever sick enough to call out and only took an occasional "mental health" day off. We all did, now and then, and a friend of mine from 9 used to call in and say, "I'm having trouble with my eyes. I can't see myself coming in today." My sentence will now be shortened by thirteen months.

"Analysis, Spock."

"He can retire in two years, three months, twenty-five days, fourteen hours, and seven minutes, Jim."

"Warp speed, Mr. Scott."

Number One—The Retirement Home?

My transfer to Paramedic 1 came through a few months later. One was located in the little town of Galesville, which was situated on the West River. This was truly rural South County or, more affectionately known as SoCo, to the locals there. There are two waterfront restaurants, a couple of marinas, an ice house, community hall, church, post office, an elementary school, and a "Mom and Pop" market, all on two streets. If you blink while you're driving by, you'll miss it. Station 1, too, was a volly company with one or two active members that never rode and an administrative board. It was an old, single-story station with four bays, facing Main Street and two in the back that made a drive-thru. It housed an engine, squad, brush truck and utility pickup along with the medic unit. It was quiet—peaceful, actually. There was a problem, though.

There were only four of us—an engineman, a firefighter, a paramedic lieutenant, and a medic. Two people on an engine or squad was craziness. So much for the two-in, two-out, RIT policy. Even if the medic unit ran with the engine on a fire call, we'd have to wait for 9 or 42 to get there before we could do anything, and in South County, that could be a while. It wasn't like North County where you had four stations in close proximity of each other. We were spread out. Get this, if the firefighter had to take the brush truck on a call, the engineman would have to take the squad or engine on another call by himself. I mentioned something about the "driver-only" policy earlier. That's so crazy, I can't even begin to comprehend it. Another critical analogy about the department was (I'll take credit for coming up with this one) "We're circling the drain and swimmin' like a son-of-a-bitch." It was sad but true.

Most of the guys that worked in South County lived close by. The rest were put there as punishment especially if they lived out of state. If you lived fifty miles from North County, you were ninety miles from the South. There was less call volume relative to a more sparse population, for the firefighters anyway. The medic unit would find itself anywhere, at any time. We had more calls covering for 3 than we did in our first due area but the important thing was, sleep. I was getting more sleep at night here compared to none at Paramedic 3. All we needed was one transport after midnight to ruin that, though. An ALS call at 1 meant, at least a two-hour turn-around time, but I was content as I could be, all things considered.

The Countdown Is On

It was nice to be able to cook a meal for four and actually complete it. Of course, sitting down and eating it was a different story. Everyone that has ever worked for a fire department, anywhere, has one bad habit that is common amongst us all—we eat fast. We could go all day, with one or two calls, prepare a meal, serve it, and as soon as we'd sit down and take one bite, waaaaaaaaaahh. I used to say, "Those fuckers have a hidden camera in here, they have to." It didn't matter if we ate at four or seven, or ten for that matter, it was scary how often it happened. Of course, it was the medic unit that always got the call. We'd rag the hell out of the engine crew if it ever happened to them and it was funny, but didn't happen very often. I was counting the shifts until I was finished when I realized one thing—they moved slower when I did that.

I had worked as a part-time captain for a Sea Ray dealership in '02, after the charter boat I was working on in Ocean City was sold. I needed to keep my hours up for my license renewal, so I chose this path. I'd make deliveries for them and learned to teach new owners about the boats they had just purchased, then take them out and show them how not to run into shit. It was fun but it only lasted two seasons before I found out that boat sales people are just like as car sales people. I'll let you think about that one. I was back to running a different charter boat during the spring and summer months of '03 and took a friend's advice when I started my own captain's service. I liked the teaching part because there are millions of boat owners that are still trying to learn docking, maneuvering, and navigation by trial and error—mostly, by error.

I liked being my own boss, most of all. I think I have a pretty good reputation as a competent skipper, so far. Let's put it this way, my friends haven't been able to call me "Captain Crunch" yet and most of the people I've taught seem to remember me, and thank me when I see them a year later. That's a good clue and I really have dreams of, one day, being able to "fly south for the winter" and run a fishing boat in Florida, then come back home to do it here during the warmer months. If I could find one here that goes to the Caribbean for the winter, I'd be set. You have to dream, folks, and I made a promise to Michael, and myself, that I would be here for him until he graduates from high school in '08. I'm already missing him and he hasn't even taken his SAT's yet.

My Last Hoorah

When I went to work for Baltimore City, I got my first letter of commendation two months after I started. I got my *last* letter of commendation two months after I moved to Paramedic 1. It was during the Blizzard of 2003.

Waaaaaaaaahh…

"Medical Box 41-04. Ambulance 41 and Paramedic 1 respond for trouble breathing at number 4120 Caraway Road, cross street, Shady Side Road." Needless to say, it was snowing its ass off. We were getting about an inch-an-hour and it had been snowing for about eight hours. My partner was Jethro, a fairly new medic who I jokingly called "My Idiot." Actually he was very smart, very young, and couldn't decide what he wanted to be, a medic or a firefighter. He was a medic tonight, whether he wanted to be or not. We plowed our way towards the scene and the snow had doubled our response time. Ambulance 41 arrived a couple of minutes before us and gave us this info.

"Ambulance 41 to Paramedic 1."

"Paramedic 1."

"We have a Priority 1 patient."

"Paramedic 1 copy, ETA five to ten." We arrived and found an elderly gentleman suffering from CHF (congestive heart failure). Many times, if you suffer a heart attack that does damage to your heart muscles, you develop this condition. Sometimes it develops naturally from old age and a lack of medical maintenance (if you are over forty, you need to get a complete physical every year, unless you like surprises).

This patient was in his seventies and had suffered from his condition for a few years, according to his wife. We responded to his distress and after placing him on high concentration oxygen and the EKG monitor, started an IV. We gave him eighty milligrams of Lasix (diuretic or fluid reducer), a sublingual (under the tongue) Nitroglycerin, which would open his blood vessels, and two milligrams of morphine, which would decrease his anxiety and ease his respiratory effort. We loaded him into the unit. His wife asked if she could ride along with us.

"Of course," I said. We'd never expect her to drive in these conditions and would have asked first, if she hadn't. Jethro got her seated in the front seat then joined me in the back of the unit. Frank, the senior firefighter from Ambulance 41, would drive us to the hospital. A thirty-minute drive to Anne Arundel General would take us an hour tonight and Frank did a great job getting us there. You recall Frank from Station 5. I first met him on the call, where we had to tear the door apart for the five-hundred pound guy when I was just a probie.

We were on a hose line together at 5, and he was acting engineman at 5 on a *big* fire at a construction company, while we were there together. His wife was a nurse and he was a geek, but I liked him, and sent them a Christmas card every year.

The elderly gentleman passed on two weeks later, but his wife sent us a wonderful letter, which earned us a letter of commendation from the chief. She praised us for our compassion, professionalism, and teamwork.

"I couldn't believe how quickly and professionally they worked during this terrible weather. I felt secure and relieved with them in my presence and appreciated their compassion for their jobs. I knew that my husband was getting the best care he could possibly get," she wrote.

It may sound trivial to you, but it was one of the greatest letters I ever received and it was the last I'd ever receive. How fitting.

My Last Flight

Working in the South meant flying with the State Police more often, too. My last flight with them was one to remember.

Waaaaaaaaahh…

"Rescue Box 42-16, Engine and Ambulance 42, Squad and Paramedic 1, EMS 3 and Battalion Chief 3, respond for an auto accident with entrapment at Route 258 and Old Sudley Road."

It was a nasty Friday night, just before midnight. We experienced a hard, wind-driven rain while en route. Engine 42 arrived and a short time later called for an additional medic unit and med-evac. I doubted if they were going to be flying in this crappy weather but protocol made us go through the motions before we would get a yea or nay.

When we arrived we found a conversion van with a family on board off the shoulder of the road. It had been t-boned on the driver's side by a work van that was sitting in the middle of the intersection with heavy front-end damage. The driver of the conversion van was a male in his fifties. His wife and grandchild had minor injuries, but he was in a bad way. We had to move fast, so Jethro went to the work van and I climbed in the side door of the conversion. Paramedic 9 was the additional unit and was about ten minutes out. I needed Jethro, *badly,* because my patient had a severe head injury, a crush injury to his left side, and was unconscious. His left upper arm had a compound (open) fracture and he bled a lot from his head injury.

Paramedic 9 arrived and Jethro was free. He came to me. I couldn't do much until the guys from the engine and squad could pop the driver's door open. The driver's seat was broken which made it tough to access the patient, so I just pumped oxygen into him with the bag-valve-mask and waited. It was a task in itself. The lieutenant from the engine came over to us and shouted, "Trooper 2, fifteen minutes." Maybe it wasn't raining at Andrews Air Force Base, where they were based, but it was raining hard here. I went back to work. Jethro was in the back of our unit, setting everything up. The extrication was easy once the door was removed. We didn't bother strapping the guy to the board and were getting soaked. We supported his head, slid him onto the board, and rolled to the unit.

"I hope that bird gets here quick, this guy needs an RSI," I said to Jethro, as we hoisted the stretcher into the unit. The flight medics were the only ones performing RSI (Rapid Sequence Intubation), at the time. It was a new procedure that involved administering a new drug that stopped the patient's breathing and made intubating head trauma patients easier. This man's brain injury made him clench his mouth shut. RSI would knock him out and relax every muscle in his body, but it was tricky. You had to be good at "tubing" because if you couldn't get the tube in, you were stuck with a patient that wasn't breathing, at all. It was being field-tested by the State Police.

Jethro and I did our thing. I bagged while he placed the EKG monitor and started two IV's. I heard the familiar sound of the Dauphin helicopter outside. The back doors swung open and in climbed Mark, my favorite flight medic. I hadn't seen him for a couple of months, on the last fly-out we had, and I knew I was going with him tonight. Jethro was afraid to fly.

"Hey bro, nice night, huh?" he said to me.

"RSI, BABY, LET'S DO IT," I said to him. He just grinned at me and started pulling supplies out of his bag. Jethro got our intubation kit and tube ready for him as I started reeling off information.

"Fifties, driver, took a big hit on the left side. He's got a big-time head injury, left side chest trauma, open left humerus, and probably a pelvis. He's been out the whole time. His teeth are clenched, snoring respirations, and no lung sounds on the left side. His left pupil is blown, BP's low but not bottomed, and his (heart) rate's up. Man, he's a classic," I rambled.

Mark just nodded the whole time. Mark and I went back a few years. He was a tall, thin guy with close-cut red hair. Was he a true redhead? There was no question in my mind and I found that out the first time we met.

When I was working at 3, Brian and I ran all the way down to 41's area on a crash with entrapment and fire at three in the morning. We were the first due medic unit because 1 and 9 were both out. It took us forever to get to the call, it seemed. Forty-One is about five miles south of 1 and at least fifteen miles from 3.

It was a clusterfuck by the time we got there. The crash was on a two-lane road with no shoulder. Most secondary roads down south are like that. We had to park the medic unit fifty yards from the crash site. The equipment there was situated so we couldn't get the stretcher through the parked engines, squad, and everything else. Brian went to Ambulance 41 and I was directed to the vehicle where my patient was. She was sitting there ALONE. I went ballistic. I called for the chief in command and started reading him the riot act. They were so worried about putting out the fire in the second vehicle they weren't even attending to her, and she had a serious leg fracture. I was cursing and hollering like a madman.

I didn't care who I was dealing with or who came to assist me, I went off on them. It was totally unacceptable care (none) and could have gotten them all busted for abandonment. I let them all know that, too. It took four firefighters to carry the stretcher down into the drainage ditch and along the parked equipment to get it close to the patient. It was a good thing it wasn't raining.

"I AIN'T CARRYING THAT FUCKIN' THING. YOU NO-PARKIN' MOTHERFUCKERS CAN CARRY IT. I'VE GOT SHIT TO DO," I ranted.

They all had the fear of God in their eyes, even the chief. No one was immune and no one said a word to me. They knew I was pissed beyond being pissed. Brian had determined that the second patient was a minor injury and joined me. He didn't say anything to me, either, he just cracked up every time I yelled at somebody—and I yelled at everybody. He knew I was right.

We got the patient out of the vehicle, which had struck a large tree. She wasn't trapped but had a closed femur (upper leg and biggest bone in the body) fracture which meant we had to be very careful with her. The pain was killing her and if you're not gentle with the fracture before getting a splint on it, a bone fragment or jagged bone end could sever one of the big blood vessels in the leg. When the large vessels bleed internally its called "compartmentation" and a patient can actually bleed to death before you realize what's happened.

Trooper 2 had been summoned and was on the ground for so long, they shut the engines down. We finally got the splint on the patient and all the advanced life support done and headed for the abandoned airfield where Trooper 2 was waiting. The pilot fired the jets up as we arrived at the LZ. Then I met poor Mark, as he climbed in the back.

"What took you guys so long?" he snapped. I don't have to tell you what happened next. Brian ran for the hills.

"YOU WANNA KNOW? YOU REALLY WANNA KNOW?" I barked. Mark was no different than the rest of them and I went off on him, too. By the time we opened the back doors and got out we were nose-to-nose, yelling at each other. I was telling him to get the poor woman to the hospital and he was lambasting me for blaming him for a bunch of incompetents. Brian and three firefighters loaded the woman into the bird. After a few last, "fuck you's," and a couple more "fuck you, too's," we finally parted company.

I saw Mark on a call a few weeks later and shamefully apologized. He did the same as we shook hands, laughed, and gave each other a hug. We've been brothers from that day on. Looking back, I get a good laugh out of it, and if Mark reads this, he will too.

Anyway, I got sidetracked—back to the story. Mark swapped places with me as I continued to breathe for the injured driver of the conversion van. He was now seated at the patient's head as I stretched the med port of the IV line to him. As he pushed the drugs, we all watched and waited. A couple of seconds later you could see the man's body "deflate," with one last breath, as the drugs kicked in. Mark opened the patient's mouth, I did a quick pass with the tip of the suction unit to clear his mouth, and the tube went in.

"Nice one, bro," I applauded. Mark slid out of the seat as I secured the tube and returned to bagging. The drug would wear off in a few minutes and it was time to fly.

"What are you doin' flying in this shit? I never expected to see ya'," I told Mark, as we rolled toward the waiting chopper.

"Yeah, well, we knew it was YOU, and you probably needed help," he said with a chuckle. Smart ass. The rain had let up some but the wind was kicking and the trees were rushing. I climbed into the jump seat of the helicopter, put the comm headset on, and buckled myself in. It was dark inside the bird but I had done this many times before. Mark followed and plugged the comm wire to his helmet. The pilot could now communicate with both of us.

"We gotta go, you ready?" I heard him say.

"Roger, get us there," Mark replied. I was nervous because I had never flown with them in bad weather. When the pilot said, "We gotta go," I got a little anxious. The chopper rocked like a boat as we lifted off.

"Hey bro, we're not gonna be able to bring you back," Mark advised me. I reached up and pinched my mic button.

"Brother, you get me THERE in one piece and I'll be happy with that. I'll walk home if I have to," I returned. I heard them both laugh. The visibility was bad with a low ceiling for flying. I thought about power lines, cell phone towers, and things we could run into, and then I decided I'd concentrate on the patient more. I took a deep breath and remembered I was flying with the best of the best. The conditions improved a little as we got closer to the hospital. It was my bumpiest ride I'd ever experienced with them and landing was a real treat, too—Rock and roll, baby. Normally, I loved flying, but I didn't like this one. It would be my last one, and the last time I'd see Mark. I miss that skinny fucker.

Paramedic 9 was transporting the man's wife and granddaughter to the same hospital, as a precaution, due to the "mechanism of injury." They would be my ride home. Our patient died a short time after we left the hospital. The driver that struck him had been at a bar since Happy Hour, which started seven hours before the accident. I couldn't imagine having to live with that memory for the rest of my life and, you should think about him the next time you're going to drink and drive.

The End

I had been diagnosed with high blood pressure about eight years ago and prescribed medication but, other than that, I was a healthy forty-eight. My mom and Dad had a history of it and it was probably gonna be there, even without the stressful environment associated with my job. Regardless, I'm in good shape, give blood every two months, and always have my yearly physical. I hate surprises. About three months before my "parole" date, I had an event.

It was a Sunday evening and we had just finished a meal of fried chicken, mashed potatoes, gravy, green beans, and fresh dinner rolls. Incredibly, I was able to prepare the entire meal, and eat it, without interruption. We all over-ate and as the five of us sat at the table, gloating, the side door of the station opened and in walked our quality assurance officer. He was the most unskilled, incompetent, advanced life support provider I had ever seen, known, or even heard of. I actually witnessed his blunders the few times I worked with him on a unit. Now he's in a position to criticize and evaluate someone's skills. That was like putting an epileptic on a bomb disposal squad. I'm not even going to give a clue as to his name, or anything—enough said.

He was what we referred to as a "No Drive," too. He'd throw you around in the back of the unit on calls, and had so many accidents on his record it wasn't funny. He was a rolling accident looking for a place to happen, yet was still able to drive fire department vehicles under emergency conditions. Normally, you're allowed one accident (depending on the severity) and if you have two within one year, it's off to fire department "driving school" before you get your driving privileges returned. (I'm surprised they didn't make him a driving instructor. It would make as much sense as the position he was in now.) He walked in, leaned against the stove next to me, and crossed his arms.

"I need to talk to you, when you finish eating," he spat. I just looked down at the empty plate in front of me and looked back at him. I was full but felt like loading another plate up just to make him wait.

"I think I'm done," I returned. I followed him into the small, paramedic office and he shut the door behind me.

"We have a problem with a call you had last shift," he scolded. I knew what call it was because it was the only call we had last shift.

"Who's we?" I asked, calmly. He never answered the question, so I knew it was just his problem. The call went like this.

Jethro and I had gotten dispatched to a home at one in the morning, for trouble breathing. We were met in the driveway by a retired firefighter who had initiated the call. The patient was his mother and he, immediately, told us she was having shoulder pain and *not* trouble breathing. I assured him we would check her out and take good care of her. She was eighty-six years old and known to most of the regular medics at 1 and 3 because of her cardiac history. She actually went into cardiac arrest one night and survived it, thanks to us. On this evening she complained of right shoulder and neck pain. She said she had taken one of her nitroglycerin pills a half hour before the call, but it didn't help. When I asked her when the pain first started, I expected to hear her say, two hours ago, when she said, "TWO WEEKS AGO."

"Two weeks ago? Why did you wait till tonight to call?" I inquired.

"Well, this is the first night that I haven't been able to sleep," she said. OK, I'm no brain surgeon, but from my assessment of her, I'm very certain she's not having a cardiac problem. She had no signs or symptoms that indicated it. Her blood pressure was slightly elevated (the nitro should have lowered it), her breathing was normal, and her lungs were clear. Her heart rate was normal, and the rhythm was regular. She was pink, warm, dry, and just didn't look like she was having a heart problem. Remember that this is not the first patient I have ever seen. I suspected an orthopedic problem so I asked the vollies on Ambulance 2, if they were comfortable taking her to the ER.

"No problem," said the younger of the two vollies. He was the aidman that would ride in the back with her and the crew chief that night. His driver was a whiny little man who was a paid man in a different department. He wanted to go back to the station and sleep and I knew this when he asked, "Shouldn't YOU take her? She took a nitroglycerin." Why do I have to justify my decision to this little man? The nitro wasn't indicated in the first place, a fucking Advil was. I can't help it if the old lady popped the wrong pill. A nitro only has an effect for a few minutes and wore off about twenty-five minutes before we even arrived.

"ARE YOU COMFORTABLE TAKING HER, OR NOT? IF NOT, I WILL," I barked. Ambulance 2 transported her without incident but that was just the start of things.

Before the QA officer showed up, today, we had been at the grocery store to buy the chicken and groceries for the Sunday meal. The guy that pushes the carts at the grocery store came up to us and told us that we had taken his grandmother to the hospital, last shift. I asked him how she was doing. He said fine, and that she had a pinched nerve in her neck. They had kept her overnight to do routine blood work because of her cardiac history. I told him that I had figured that out. I was right about her condition.

Earlier that day we had a call, and saw the crew from Paramedic 9 at the ER. One of the medics from 9 told me that he was at the hospital the night the tired little twit that drove Ambulance 2 that night, came in to the ER telling everyone, "Paramedic 1 just dumped this chest pain on us." Apparently, he had made the same claim to the QA officer, too. It was all taking shape now. I will spare you the details but I will tell you that I have never been in as heated an argument with any man, any time in my life, until this day. He's lucky I didn't punch his lights out and I actually threatened him with bodily harm if he ever second-guessed any of my patient care again. He stormed out of the building, slamming the door, as I returned to the kitchen. The captain and battalion chief that had just eaten with us just sat there, and never came in to intervene. I know they could hear us. I was still cussing him as my partner that day, Larry, looked at me. He said I was so pissed that my "eyes were red." He wanted to take my blood pressure, so I agreed.

"Yeah, your pressure's up. It's 170 over 110 and where'd you get that irregular heartbeat?" he asked. WHAT? I've never had that in my life. My EKG has always been normal for ten years. Larry told the captain to call Communications and put the medic unit out of service until he could give me an EKG, and let me cool off. We found that I was in atrial fibrillation—great, the QA asshole almost killed me! Twenty minutes later my pressure had come down, but I was still in a-fib. Paramedic 9 was summoned and took me to the ER. They did everything to me that I had been doing to people for over twenty years.

As I lay on the stretcher in the back of Paramedic 9, on my way to the hospital, I realized that my illustrious career was coming to an end. I couldn't handle the job any more and it had nothing to do with my ability to lift, drag, carry, calculate dosages, make split-second decisions, fight fire, or comfort a poor soul. I couldn't deal with the idiots or the bullshit anymore.

I was released from the ER that night but was still in a-fib. I had an appointment with a cardiologist the next day and woke up that morning, still in a-fib. I was getting worried and scared. I called the chief of EMS before my doctor's appointment and explained the circumstances surrounding the entire incident, including the call with the old lady that started the whole thing. I told him I was probably not coming back to work. He had known me for my entire career. He cussed the QA, and complained about the number of problems he was having with him. He asked me to write Special Reports documenting the events as I had just stated them to him, on the phone.

I felt better after getting his support. I hung the phone up, took a deep breath, and checked my pulse. It was normal and regular. I had broken the a-fib sometime during the conversation. I went to the cardiologist later that morning and my EKG was normal. She told me that I couldn't return to work but, somehow, I already knew that. My request for a medical retirement due to occupational heart disease, was denied by the county because there was "no proof," other than the "isolated occurrence" that night. Why wasn't I surprised? I burned some sick leave and was able to take my normal retirement, two months later, on October 1, 2004.

I haven't had a-fib since. The show is over.

The QA lieutenant is now a captain and I'm happily retired, right where I belong—living on my houseboat, teaching people safe boating, moving yachts, and fishing every chance I get. Louie, Cuz, and Alan can rest now. I finally made it home for the last time.

Epilogue

The moral of this story is, there *is* no moral. Life goes on with or without us, and it's fragile. I think that I have accomplished what the Higher Powers have put me in this world to do. I learned about life and death and used that knowledge to help those that might not understand it or be able cope with it in their time of need. I think it helped make me a better person and I know I saved a few people. My career as an Emergency Services provider spanned three-and-a-half decades. I brought life into this world eleven times but can't tell you how many times I saw it leave. I hope that you can see things a little clearer now. I hope that you can say that you've learned something from reading this. Hopefully it's something that might make your lives better or perhaps help you look at your own life in a different perspective. I've always been one to speak words of wisdom from lessons I have learned, and here are a few.

First, and foremost, keep in touch with your family, both immediate and extended. They are one of your most valuable assets and you never know when they'll be gone forever. Make contact often, even if it's for a minute, to say hi. It may do more for them than it does for you.

Second, be a role model for children. Whether you realize it or not, you're a teacher. All children learn from our actions and they are our future, and future strength of our world. Every single one is eager to learn, so teach them right from wrong, how to respect others, and most importantly, how to respect themselves.

Jim Valvano was the most inspirational person I ever saw, or heard. I wish I had the opportunity to meet him in person. For those who don't know who he was, I'll tell you.

Jimmy V was the men's basketball coach at North Carolina State University in 1993. He was fun to watch on the sidelines and listen to in post-game interviews. His intensity and love for the game was unmatched by anyone, but more important was his love for his kids. Not only did he teach them

196

the game of basketball but taught them how to win in the game of life as a role model. Not long after he and his kids realized a dream and won the NCAA Division I National Championship, he was diagnosed with cancer.

The disease was advanced and moved through his body quickly, but before he fell victim and left our world, he was honored by ESPN at their annual ESPY Awards Ceremony, as they presented him with their coveted "Arthur Ashe Courage Award." If you don't ever see another film clip as long as you live, you must see this one. His speech was the most inspirational I've ever seen, and I get choked up just thinking about it. In it he talks about his disease and the things it has taken from him, but reminds all of us that,

"....it cannot touch my mind, it cannot touch my heart, and it cannot touch my soul, and those three things are gonna carry on forever." He concluded with seven famous words that are the motto of his cancer research foundation. These words of encouragement changed how I look at death and defeat. He said, *"Don't give up...Don't EVER give up."* Thank you, Jimmy V., for your wisdom, your ethics, your beliefs, and most of all, your courage. You've touched thousands, perhaps millions, and the Jimmy V. Foundation for Cancer Research is a great honor in your memory. I'll see you on the other side one day.

If you think your life is bad and you have events that try to take away your mind, your heart, and your soul, do something about it. You are able to. Think about the words you just read and do something to make your life better, or change things—but don't give up. There are millions of people whose lives suck every day, and have since they've been on this rock. There are millions who will never get the opportunity to change their lives and wouldn't know how if they did. I know this for a fact because I've met a few of them and you've just read about them. Don't give up, don't EVER give up.

Finally, always remember to "watch your back" every day, and if you can't, find comfort in knowing that there will always be someone out there, like me, who will.

LaVergne, TN USA
13 December 2010
208651LV00004B/133/P